YOGA
TO THE RESCUE

REMEDIES FOR REAL GIRLS

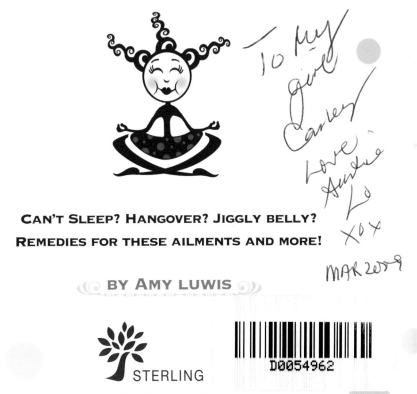

CAN'T SLEEP? HANGOVER? JIGGLY BELLY?
REMEDIES FOR THESE AILMENTS AND MORE!

BY AMY LUWIS

STERLING

New York / London
www.sterlingpublishing.com

D0054962

To My girl Carley Love Aunti Lo xox

MAR 2009

STERLING and the distinctive Sterling logo are
registered trademarks of Sterling Publishing Co., Inc.

LIBRARY OF CONGRESS CATALOGING-IN-PUBLICATION DATA AVAILABLE

2 4 6 8 10 9 7 5 3

Published in 2007 by Sterling Publishing Co., Inc.
387 Park Avenue South, New York, NY 10016
Published originally as a set of instructional cards
by Playground Press
Box 4575, Falls Church, Virginia 22044
© 2005 by Amy Luwis
Distributed in Canada by Sterling Publishing
c/o Canadian Manda Group, 165 Dufferin Street
Toronto, Ontario, Canada M6K 3H6
Distributed in the United Kingdom by GMC Distribution Services
Castle Place, 166 High Street, Lewes, East Sussex, England BN7 1XU
Distributed in Australia by Capricorn Link (Australia) Pty. Ltd.
P.O. Box 704, Windsor, NSW 2756, Australia

Sterling ISBN-13: 978-1-4027-4880-6
ISBN-10: 1-4027-4880-9

For information about custom editions, special sales, premium and
corporate purchases, please contact Sterling Special Sales
Department at 800-805-5489 or specialsales@sterlingpublishing.com.

CONTENTS

For my parents, Frank and Brenda, to whom I owe so much.

For Bryan Lewis Aspey, extraordinary guitarist and composer,
whose love, friendship, and wisdom can lighten even the darkest moments.

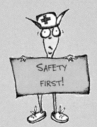

This book is *not* intended to diagnose, treat, cure, or prevent any disease
or condition. If you have a health concern or condition, consult your doctor
or health care provider. Always consult your doctor before starting
any new exercise program.

Now have some fun!

INTRODUCTION

Stressed? Tired? Plump?
In pain? Ready to drop out of society
or check into a nuthouse?

◎

If you relate to any of these ailments, then yoga is the
tonic for you. Yoga reduces stress, boosts energy and the
immune system, eliminates toxins, tones muscles, reduces
pain (physical and mental), increases confidence, and
generates clarity—really and truly!

This amazing little book is packed with 48
classic yoga poses *(asanas)* that will start you
on a journey to total wellness.

NAMASTE!

BIG STUFF

LITTLE THINGS THAT MAKE A BIG DIFFERENCE

- It's important to practice on an empty stomach so your body can focus on yoga and not digestion.

- Start by warming up your muscles. You can do this with a quick walk or by massaging your limbs or by taking a bath.

- Getting out of a pose is just as important as getting into it. Follow these general rules: Safety and comfort come first. Move slowly. Press with firm legs to come up out of standing poses. To get out of reclining poses, always roll to one side. To come out of standing or seated forward bends, lift your head only after you are fully upright.

- End your yoga workout with a relaxation pose like the corpse pose, Savasana (page 106).

- Never do inverted poses if you have a headache or during your period. On your heaviest flow days, stick to the Ragtime category (page 108).

- Never do unsupported back bends if you are pregnant, menstruating, or if you have heart problems or other serious physical conditions.

- If you have knee, back, or neck problems, practice with an experienced teacher.

Hints: Back bends combat depression. Forward bends calm nerves. Standing poses increase emotional stability and strength. Inverted poses boost energy.

SINK or SEQUENCE

At the beginning of each category you'll find Mega Benefit Sequences that boost the benefits in that particular category. For instance, are you really stressed? Then do a Calm Mega Benefit Sequence, not just a single pose from the Calm category. A good general rule—the benefits from any yoga workout increase if you do a sequence of poses.

The order in which you sequence poses will depend on your needs and state of mind at the time. Really listen to your body, and soon you'll be able to tailor your routines to your specific needs. By practicing yoga regularly you'll also learn how long you can comfortably stay in a pose, and you'll begin to notice the benefits of each pose and sequence.

There are no strict rules governing the order in which you do these poses, but some general principles can be used to make the poses more effective together.

Here is a basic sequence:
1. Standing pose
2. Back bend
3. Forward bend
4. Twisting pose
5. Inversion
6. Restorative pose

Hint: A good way to learn sequencing is to follow routines arranged by an experienced yoga instructor.

IN THE KNOW

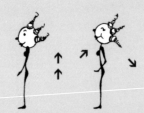

Breathing: The essence of yoga—and the key to relaxation—is proper breathing. Learn to be mindful of your breathing, and practice breathing deeply and steadily. Never hold your breath! (This is common when attempting a difficult pose.)

Find your sit bones: When doing any sitting poses, it is important to center yourself on your sit bones. To locate them, sit up straight on a hard surface. Place a hand under each side of your derriere, and draw the flesh away from the bone. You should feel your sit bones pressing into the floor. Distribute your weight evenly between them.

Roll your shoulders: Rolling your shoulders back is one of the best things you can do for good posture. Start by lifting your shoulders up as if you were shrugging (as the girl on the left is doing). Now roll your shoulders back, pressing your shoulder blades into your body and lifting your chest.

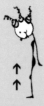

Lift your kneecaps: Lifting your kneecaps by tightening your thighs may sound odd, but it works and it's really good for your knees and legs. Try it standing in front of a mirror; tighten your thigh muscles just above your knees, and you should see your kneecaps lift up.

*A yogini is a female yoga practitioner.

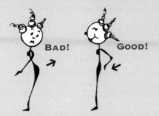

Your tailbone: Where is it? Your tailbone is at the very end of your spine. Many people swing it back, which puts pressure on your lower back. Always try to bring your tailbone forward, especially when practicing standing poses. Doing so will protect your back and keep it strong. *Don't* bring your entire lower back forward—that's a common mistake.

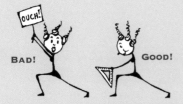

The degree of your knee: Don't bend your knee beyond 90°. You will cause unnecessary stress to your knee, like "ouch" girl above. The best way to keep your knee at 90° is NEVER to extend it beyond your ankle.

Find your crown: It's not the tiara we all dream of wearing, but it's an important part of your head that's used in certain yoga poses (the headstand, in particular). The girl at the left is wearing a beret on her crown. Your crown is at the top back of your head.

Open your chest: This is one of the most effective mood-lifters around. Imagine your chest being lifted into the sky by a balloon. Rolling your shoulders back increases the lift.

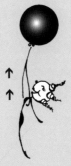

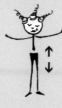

Lift your waist off your hips: Not literally! Imagine your waist and hips being pulled apart like taffy—waist up, hips down!

ACCESSORIZE

Enhancing your yoga workout with practical props helps you achieve great results. Some of the props you'll want before getting started are: a metal folding chair, a blanket, a bolster, a strap, several wooden blocks, and a sticky mat. If you don't have some of these items, be creative and use what you have at home—a sturdy chair with a hard seat, a phone book (about 5 inches thick) instead of a block, or a firm pillow or couch cushion in place of a bolster.

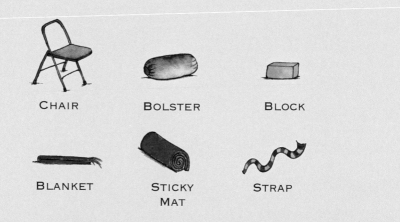

CHAIR   BOLSTER   BLOCK

BLANKET   STICKY MAT   STRAP

Even if you do yoga in a windowless basement with only your cat as an audience, wear something that's comfortable and makes you feel good about yourself. This will help you have a positive attitude and fuel your desire to practice yoga.

GETTING STARTED

The poses in this book are separated into seven color-coded categories (see below). Two pages are devoted to each pose. The first page is a detailed drawing of a real girl who is fully in the pose. Instructions for an *Easier Pose* are also included on this page in the upper right-hand corner. Don't be discouraged even if you are unable to do the *Easier Pose*. People who have been practicing yoga for years continually work on improving their poses. Remember, the goal is progress, not perfection. The first page for each pose is labeled with its name in both Sanskrit (the classical language of India) and its Western translation. This facing page provides a step-by-step list of instructions on how to get into the pose yourself (how to do it with style) and a list of other benefits—both mental and physical—as well as focus points to help you achieve the correct pose and receive all its benefits.

- **SEXY:** FITNESS & CONFIDENCE
- **CALM:** STRESS RELIEF
- **ENERGY:** BOOST & INVIGORATE
- **RESTORE:** FEEL LIKE A KID AGAIN
- **CLEANSE:** DETOX & PURIFY
- **SANITY:** MOOD & BALANCE
- **RAGTIME:** PMS & PERIOD RELIEF

◎ ◎ ◎ ◎ ◎ ◎ ◎ ◎ ◎

Hints:
Choose a category you'd like to work on and do a few poses, or do a Mega Benefit Sequence from the beginning of the category.

Have a headache? Do pose 20. Are you bloated? Do pose 35. Can't sleep? Do pose 29, and so on.

Are you stressed at work? Take a yoga break instead of a coffee break and do a Calm pose every day. Invite your co-workers and together start melting away the collective stress!

QUICK REFERENCE

SEXY: FITNESS & CONFIDENCE

1. Utkatasana (chair pose): gives you buns of steel
2. Utthita Hasta Padasana (extended hand & foot pose): increases overall strength
3. Parsva Hasta Padasana (extended side hand & foot pose): increases overall strength
4. Virabhadrasana II (warrior pose 2): firms thighs
5. Padangusthasana (foot & big toe pose): improves posture
6. Parsvottanasana (intense side stretch pose): opens chest
7. Gomukhasana (cow face pose—arms only): loosens shoulders
8. Chaturanga Dandasana (four limb staff pose): firms tummy
9. Parivrtta Trikonasana (revolving triangle pose): firms calves
10. Urdhva Prasarita Padasana (upward extended foot pose): firms middle

CALM: STRESS RELIEF

11. Adho Mukha Virasana (child's pose): relieves tension
12. Adho Mukha Svanasana (downward facing dog pose): relieves anger
13. Prasarita Padottanasana I (extended leg intense stretch pose 1): calms anxious nerves
14. Ardha Chandrasana (half moon pose): improves balance
15. Urdhva Mukha Svanasana (upward facing dog pose): releases pent-up energy

ENERGY: BOOST & INVIGORATE

16. Tadasana (mountain pose): perks you up!
17. Urdhva Hastasana (upward hand pose): releases tension in upper back
18. Vrksasana (tree pose): improves balance
19. Dandasana (staff pose): stimulates respiratory system
20. Prasarita Padottanasana (extended leg intense stretch pose): relieves tension headache
21. Virabhadrasana III (warrior pose 3): invigorates the entire body
22. Dhanurasana (bow pose): loosens joints and improves mobility

RESTORE: FEEL LIKE A KID AGAIN

23. Paschima Namaskarasana (back body prayer pose): invigorates hands, wrists, and shoulders
24. Virasana (hero pose): soothes and strengthens knees
25. Paschimottanasana (intense stretch of the west pose): quiets the monkey mind!
26. Supta Padangusthasana I (reclined big toe pose 1): soothes a sore back
27. Utthita Trikonasana (extended triangle pose): invigorates circulation
28. Utthita Parsvakonasana (extended side angle pose): relieves sciatica and back pain
29. Halasana (plough pose): reduces insomnia
30. Salamba Sirsasana (headstand pose): improves memory and alertness
31. Salamba Sarvangasana (shoulder stand pose): soothes frazzled nerves

CLEANSE: DETOX & PURIFY

32. Baddhakonasana (bound angle pose): alleviates a full tummy
33. Uttanasana (intense forward stretch pose): soothes a hangover
34. Marichyasana I (Marichi's pose 1): tones and detoxifies organs
35. Paripurna Navasana (full boat pose): eliminates gas and bloating
36. Bharadvajasana (Bharadvaja's pose): realigns the spine
37. Bharadvajasana I (Bharadvaja's pose 1): refreshes and enlivens

SANITY: MOOD & BALANCE

38. Upavistha Konasana (seated wide angle pose): improves libido
39. Virabhadransana I (warrior pose 1): increases confidence
40. Ustrasana (camel pose): lifts your spirits and relieves depression
41. Urdhva Dhanurasana (upward facing bow pose): improves your mood and relieves depression
42. Viparita Karani (inverted lake pose): soothes and restores
43. Savasana (corpse pose): brings tranquility and peace

RAGTIME: PMS & PERIOD RELIEF

44. Supta Baddha Konasana (reclining bound angle pose): improves clarity and focus
45. Supta Virasana (reclined hero's pose): reduces appetite
46. Adho Muhka Baddakonasana (downward facing bound angle pose): alleviates hormonal tears
47. Paschimottanasana (intense stretch pose): improves grounding
48. Sukasana (cross-legged pose): empties the mind and creates inner harmony

SEXY

FITNESS & CONFIDENCE

Sexy isn't about how your backside looks

in a pair of jeans.

Sexy is about self-confidence and self-acceptance.

The beauty of yoga is it works ALL your muscles,

stretching and strengthening each one—including

your mind muscle—and gives you a feeling of

empowerment and peace.

Now, that's sexy!

MEGA BENEFIT SEQUENCES

THE NUMBERS BELOW RESCUEGIRL CORRESPOND TO THE POSES.

SEQUENCE 1

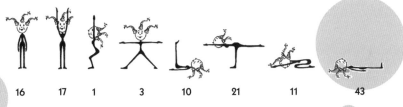

| 16 | 17 | 1 | 3 | 10 | 21 | 11 | 43 |

SEQUENCE 2

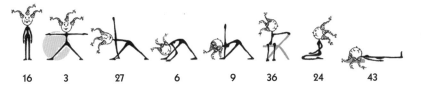

| 16 | 3 | 27 | 6 | 9 | 36 | 24 | 43 |

SEQUENCE 3

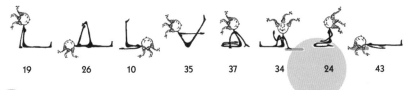

| 19 | 26 | 10 | 35 | 37 | 34 | 24 | 43 |

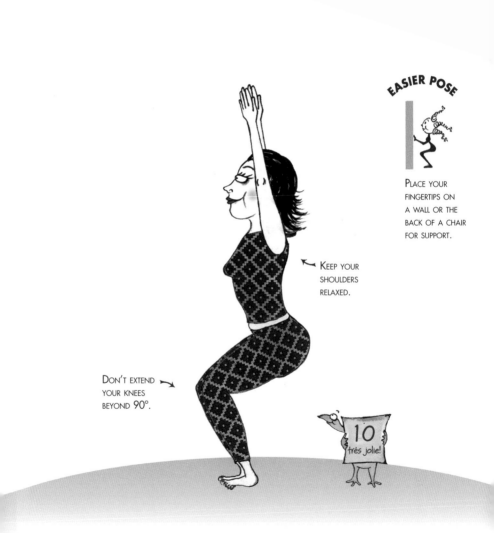

EASIER POSE

PLACE YOUR
FINGERTIPS ON
A WALL OR THE
BACK OF A CHAIR
FOR SUPPORT.

KEEP YOUR
SHOULDERS
RELAXED.

DON'T EXTEND
YOUR KNEES
BEYOND 90°.

10
très jolie!

How to do it with style!

1 Stand up straight with your feet together.

2 Stretch your arms strongly over your head.

3 Roll your shoulders back and lift your chest.

4 Slowly bend your knees.

5 Keep your heels firmly on the floor.

6 Deepen the position.

HOLD FOR 30 SECONDS.
REPEAT A FEW MORE TIMES.

Other benefits

Increases overall strength
and endurance •
Strengthens tummy, thighs,
and back

Focus points

As you deepen the bend
of the knees, maintain a
straight line from
the top of your head
to your tailbone.

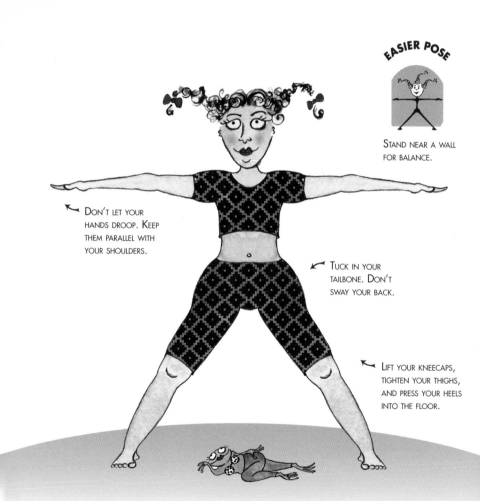

STAND NEAR A WALL
FOR BALANCE.

DON'T LET YOUR
HANDS DROOP. KEEP
THEM PARALLEL WITH
YOUR SHOULDERS.

TUCK IN YOUR
TAILBONE. DON'T
SWAY YOUR BACK.

LIFT YOUR KNEECAPS,
TIGHTEN YOUR THIGHS,
AND PRESS YOUR HEELS
INTO THE FLOOR.

Does zipping your jeans cause oxygen deprivation? This helps you breathe.

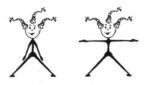

How to do it with style!

1 Stand with your legs wide apart.

2 Raise your arms to shoulder height.

3 Lift your kneecaps to tighten your thighs.

4 Bring your tailbone in.

5 Roll your shoulders back and lift your chest.

6 Look straight ahead.

HOLD FOR **1–3** MINUTES.

Other benefits

Strengthens your ankles and legs • Tones your tummy, back, and chest

Focus points

Keep your weight evenly distributed and your feet firmly anchored on the ground.

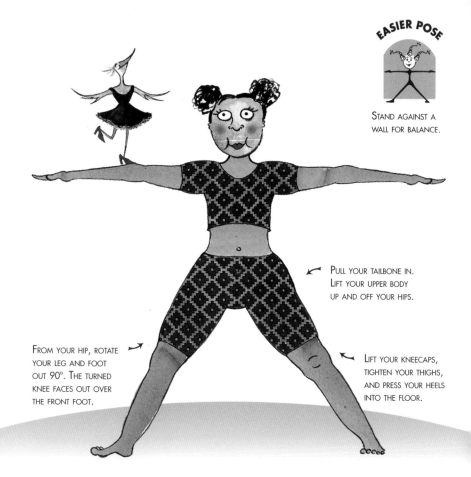

EASIER POSE

STAND AGAINST A
WALL FOR BALANCE.

PULL YOUR TAILBONE IN.
LIFT YOUR UPPER BODY
UP AND OFF YOUR HIPS.

FROM YOUR HIP, ROTATE
YOUR LEG AND FOOT
OUT 90°. THE TURNED
KNEE FACES OUT OVER
THE FRONT FOOT.

LIFT YOUR KNEECAPS,
TIGHTEN YOUR THIGHS,
AND PRESS YOUR HEELS
INTO THE FLOOR.

Want to get back into that favorite dress? This helps you get into shape.

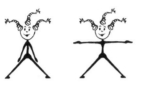

How to do it with style!

1 Stand with your legs a comfortable width apart.

2 Raise your arms to shoulder height.

3 Lift your kneecaps by tightening your thighs.

4 Bring your tailbone in.

5 Keep your torso and hips facing forward.

6 Turn your right foot out 90° and turn your left toes in slightly.

7 Roll your shoulders back and lift your chest.

8 Look straight ahead.

HOLD FOR **1–3** MINUTES.
REPEAT ON THE OTHER SIDE.

Other benefits

Strengthens ankles, knees, and hips • Tones arms and upper back • Improves balance

Focus points

Keep your hips, chest, and shoulders facing forward. Keep your arms and legs straight and strong.

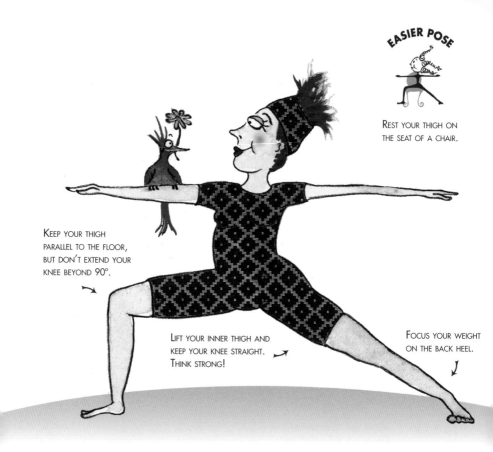

EASIER POSE

Rest your thigh on the seat of a chair.

Keep your thigh parallel to the floor, but don't extend your knee beyond 90°.

Lift your inner thigh and keep your knee straight. Think strong!

Focus your weight on the back heel.

Wobbly thighs?
This will make them strong and firm.

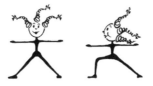

How to do it with style!

1 Stand with your legs a comfortable distance apart.

2 Raise your arms to shoulder height.

3 Lift your kneecaps by tightening your thighs.

4 Bring your tailbone in.

5 Turn your right foot out to 90° and turn your left toes in slightly.

6 Roll your shoulders back and lift your chest.

7 Bend your right knee to 90°.

8 Keep your torso and hips facing forward.

9 Lift your waist up and off your hips.

10 Turn your head and look over your right arm.

HOLD FOR **30** SECONDS.
REPEAT ON THE OTHER SIDE.

Other benefits

Increases flexibility of hips • Strengthens legs • Encourages determination

Focus points

This pose requires lots of energy, so breathe deeply. Maintain strong limbs.

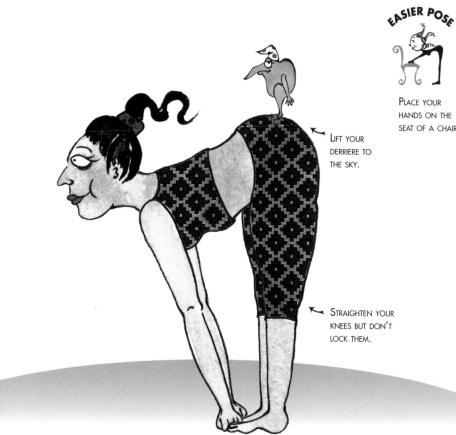

PLACE YOUR
HANDS ON THE
SEAT OF A CHAIR.

LIFT YOUR
DERRIERE TO
THE SKY.

STRAIGHTEN YOUR
KNEES BUT DON'T
LOCK THEM.

Does the Hunchback of Notre Dame have
better posture? This will help
you straighten up.

5
SEXY

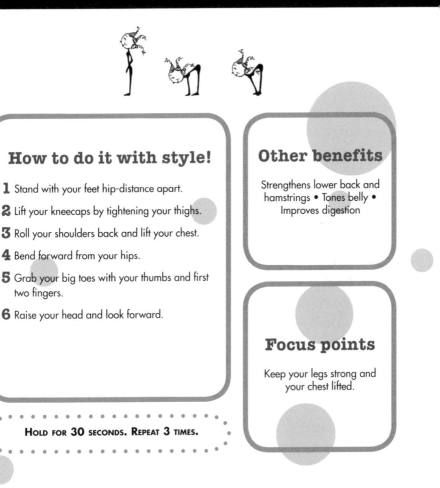

How to do it with style!

1 Stand with your feet hip-distance apart.

2 Lift your kneecaps by tightening your thighs.

3 Roll your shoulders back and lift your chest.

4 Bend forward from your hips.

5 Grab your big toes with your thumbs and first two fingers.

6 Raise your head and look forward.

HOLD FOR **30** SECONDS. REPEAT **3** TIMES.

Other benefits

Strengthens lower back and hamstrings • Tones belly • Improves digestion

Focus points

Keep your legs strong and your chest lifted.

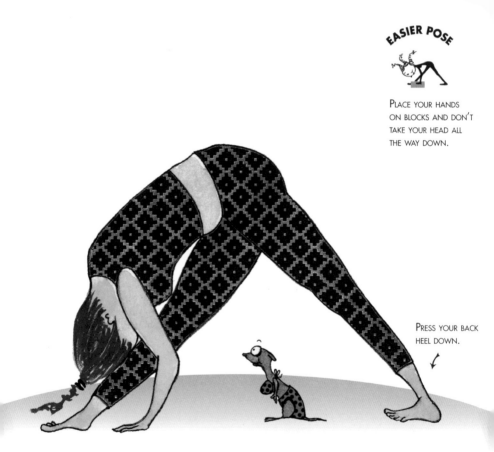

PLACE YOUR HANDS
ON BLOCKS AND DON'T
TAKE YOUR HEAD ALL
THE WAY DOWN.

PRESS YOUR BACK
HEEL DOWN.

Does your chest resemble a sunken soufflé? This will help you open up.

6
SEXY

  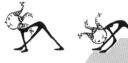

How to do it with style!

1 Stand with your legs a comfortable distance apart.

2 Lift your kneecaps by tightening your thighs.

3 Put your hands on your hips.

4 Turn your right foot out 90° and turn your left toes slightly in.

5 Turn your torso so it's facing over your right leg.

6 Bend forward from your hips and lift your chest.

7 Move your torso forward and down over your thigh.

8 Place your palms on the floor by your ankles.

9 Rest your head on your shin if you can.

HOLD FOR **30** SECONDS.
REPEAT ON THE OTHER SIDE.

Other benefits

Improves droopy shoulders • Loosens stiff hips and hamstrings • Calms mind and body

Focus points

Make sure your legs are in line, as if you're standing on a balance beam.

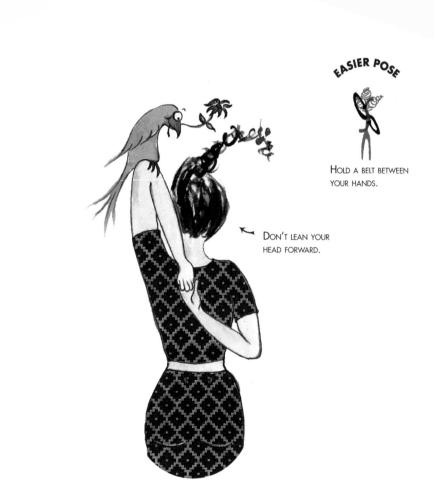

HOLD A BELT BETWEEN
YOUR HANDS.

DON'T LEAN YOUR
HEAD FORWARD.

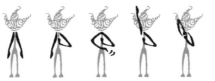

How to do it with style!

1 Bend your right elbow and swing it to the back.

2 Place the top of your right hand on your lower back.

3 Push your right hand up between your shoulder blades with your left hand.

4 Raise your left arm.

5 Bend your left elbow and rest your hand between your shoulder blades.

6 Clasp the fingers of both hands together.

Other benefits

Removes stiffness in shoulders • Opens the chest • Reduces lung congestion

Focus points

Keep your upper elbow pointing straight up. Keep your chest open.

HOLD FOR **30** SECONDS–**1** MINUTE.
REPEAT ON THE OTHER SIDE.

ANCHOR YOUR TOES ON THE
FLOOR, AND PLACE A BOLSTER
UNDER YOUR HIPS.

DON'T RAISE YOUR
BUTTOCKS.

LIFT YOUR HIPS, THIGHS,
AND KNEES OFF THE FLOOR.

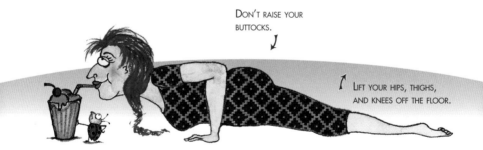

Having a love affair with ice cream?
This helps tone your tummy.

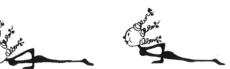

How to do it with style!

1 Lie on your stomach and rest your forehead on the floor.

2 Bend your elbows and place your palms by your sides (index fingers in line with your chest).

3 Press your palms and feet firmly into the floor.

4 Lift your legs, hips, chest, and head off the floor.

5 Keep your elbows close to your ribs.

6 Keep your butt in line with your shoulders and heels.

7 Face forward.

HOLD FOR **5–10** SECONDS. REPEAT **3** TIMES.

Other benefits

Strengthens upper body, arms, and wrists • Increases stamina • Invigorates the mind and body

Focus points

Maintain strong arms and legs to support your torso. Keep your ankles and feet strong.

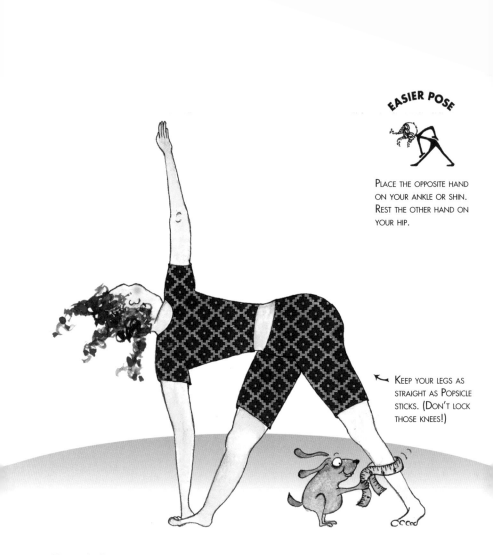

EASIER POSE

PLACE THE OPPOSITE HAND ON YOUR ANKLE OR SHIN. REST THE OTHER HAND ON YOUR HIP.

KEEP YOUR LEGS AS STRAIGHT AS POPSICLE STICKS. (DON'T LOCK THOSE KNEES!)

How to do it with style!

1 Stand with legs a comfortable distance apart.

2 Put your hands on your hips.

3 Turn your right foot out 90° and turn your left toes slightly in.

4 Turn your torso toward your right leg.

5 Raise your arms out to shoulder height.

6 Reach your left arm forward, rotating your torso to the right.

7 Place your left fingertips on floor by your right little toe.

8 Straighten your legs.

9 Extend the spine, lift your chest, and rotate a little more.

10 Lift your right arm up in line with your shoulder.

11 Turn your head upward and look toward the sky.

HOLD FOR **15** SECONDS.
REPEAT ON THE OTHER SIDE.

Other benefits

Slims your waist • Relieves back tension • Stimulates the kidneys • Improves digestion

Focus points

Keep your legs strong and anchor them firmly on the ground. Focus on lengthening and twisting your spine.

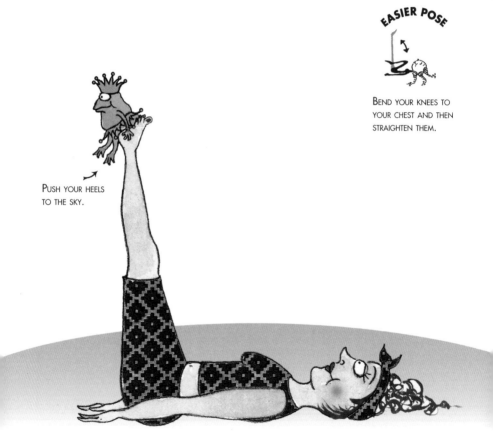

EASIER POSE

BEND YOUR KNEES TO YOUR CHEST AND THEN STRAIGHTEN THEM.

PUSH YOUR HEELS TO THE SKY.

Do you have the waistline of a toad?
This helps whittle your middle.

**10
SEXY**

How to do it with style!

1 Lie on your back with your legs stretched out.

2 Press palms down next to your sides.

3 Bend your knees and bring them to your chest.

4 Lift your feet up and straighten your legs.

5 Push your heels to the sky.

Other benefits

Tones your lower back and abdominals • Strengthens your spine • Relieves bloating and gas

Focus points

Maintain strong legs. Open your chest. Press your lower spine into the floor.

HOLD FOR **30** SECONDS–**1** MINUTE.
REPEAT **3** TIMES.

CALM

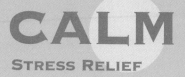

STRESS RELIEF

Yoga has all the key
elements to help you relax your body,
calm your mind, and soothe your
nervous system.

This strong foundation will help you face
life's challenges with a
peaceful mind and a calm heart!

MEGA BENEFIT SEQUENCES

The numbers below RescueGirl correspond to the poses.

Sequence 1

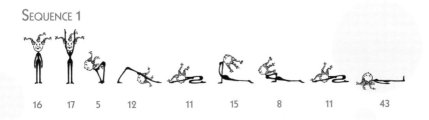

16   17   5   12   11   15   8   11   43

Sequence 2

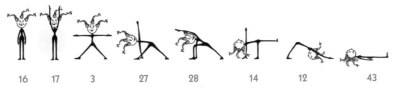

16   17   3   27   28   14   12   43

Sequence 3

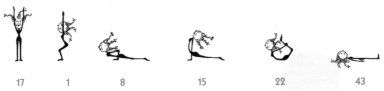

17   1   8   15   22   43

Adho Mukha Virasana
(child's pose)

EASIER POSE

PLACE A FOLDED BLANKET UNDER YOUR HEAD. PUT A ROLLED-UP BLANKET UNDER YOUR ANKLES.

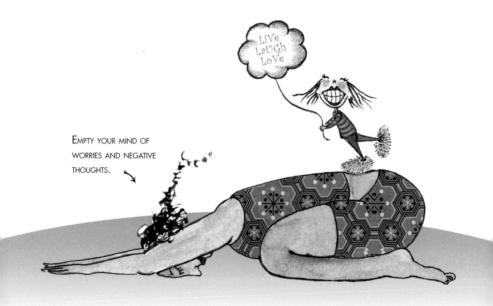

EMPTY YOUR MIND OF WORRIES AND NEGATIVE THOUGHTS.

Misplaced your inner child?
This helps melt tension so you can find her.

How to do it with style!

1 Start on your hands and knees.

2 Place your knees hip-distance apart and keep your feet together.

3 Lean back and sit on your heels.

4 Extend your arms and torso forward.

5 Rest your forehead on the floor.

6 Stretch your arms out in front of you.

7 Press your palms into the floor and your buttocks into your heels.

HOLD FOR 1–5 MINUTES.

Other benefits

Calms nerves • Lowers blood pressure • Releases tension in your neck, back, and shoulders

Focus points

Stretch out your back. Relax your neck.

Adho Mukha Svanasana
(downward facing dog pose)

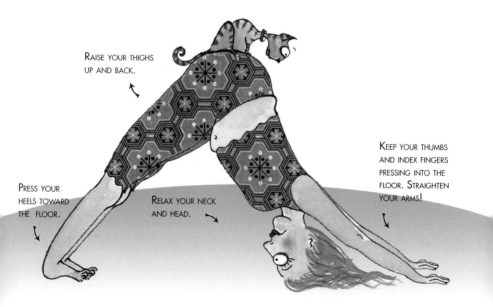

EASIER POSE

PLACE YOUR PALMS ON THE SEAT OF A CHAIR.

RAISE YOUR THIGHS UP AND BACK.

PRESS YOUR HEELS TOWARD THE FLOOR.

RELAX YOUR NECK AND HEAD.

KEEP YOUR THUMBS AND INDEX FINGERS PRESSING INTO THE FLOOR. STRAIGHTEN YOUR ARMS!

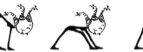 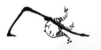

How to do it with style!

1 Place your palms on the floor in front of you.

2 Step your legs back one at a time.

3 Place your feet in line with your hands.

4 Spread your fingers and press your palms down.

5 Stretch your arms forward, keeping your elbows straight.

6 Raise your butt up to the sky and move your thighs up and back.

7 Lower your heels to the floor with your feet pointing straight ahead.

8 Relax your head and the back of your neck.

HOLD FOR **30** SECONDS–**1** MINUTE.

Other benefits

Relieves depression •
Increases the flexibility of
your hips, knees, and ankles
• Calms your mind

Focus points

Keep your legs firm and
your elbows straight as you
lift your derriere to the sky!

Prasarita Padottanasana I
(extended leg intense stretch pose 1)

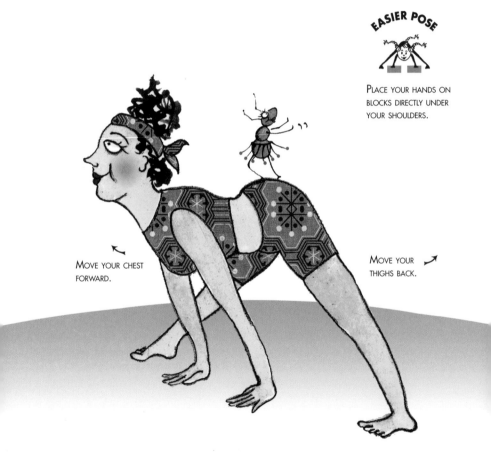

EASIER POSE

Place your hands on blocks directly under your shoulders.

Move your chest forward.

Move your thighs back.

Got ants in your pants?
This helps calm anxious nerves.

How to do it with style!

1 Stand with your legs a comfortable width apart.

2 Put your hands on your hips.

3 Stretch your torso forward and put your hands on the floor.

4 Lift your kneecaps by tightening your thighs.

5 Keep your legs straight and move your thighs back.

6 Lift your chest and head.

7 Look straight ahead.

HOLD FOR 30 SECONDS–1 MINUTE.

Other benefits

Relieves mental and physical stress • Energizes your legs • Tones your uterus

Focus points

Keep your legs firm and straight and your neck and shoulders relaxed.

Ardha Chandrasana
(half moon pose)

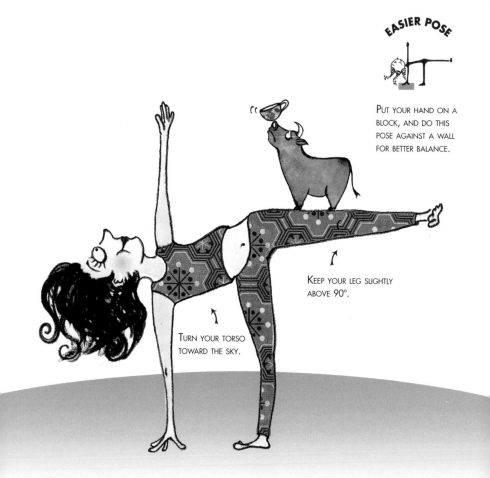

EASIER POSE

PUT YOUR HAND ON A BLOCK, AND DO THIS POSE AGAINST A WALL FOR BETTER BALANCE.

KEEP YOUR LEG SLIGHTLY ABOVE 90°.

TURN YOUR TORSO TOWARD THE SKY.

Clumsier than a bull in a china shop?
This helps improve your balance.

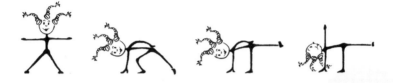

How to do it with style!

1 Stand with your legs a comfortable width apart.

2 Raise your arms to shoulder height.

3 Lift your kneecaps by tightening your thighs.

4 Bring your tailbone in.

5 Turn your right foot out 90° and turn your left toes slightly in.

6 Keep your torso and hips facing forward.

7 As you bend your right knee, lean your torso forward and place your right hand on the floor.

8 Lift your left leg up to slightly above 90°.

9 Straighten your right leg.

10 Stretch your left arm up and look up at your hand.

HOLD FOR **15** SECONDS.
REPEAT ON THE OTHER SIDE.

Other benefits

Combats fatigue • Reduces heavy menstrual bleeding and PMS • Alleviates morning sickness

Focus points

Keep your chest and hips forward. Don't let the lifted leg droop.

Urdhva Mukha Svanasana
(upward facing dog pose)

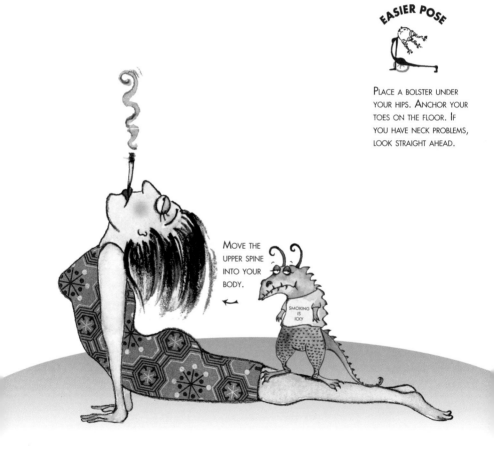

EASIER POSE

PLACE A BOLSTER UNDER YOUR HIPS. ANCHOR YOUR TOES ON THE FLOOR. IF YOU HAVE NECK PROBLEMS, LOOK STRAIGHT AHEAD.

MOVE THE UPPER SPINE INTO YOUR BODY.

SMOKING IS ICKY

Are you fuming with frustration?
This helps release pent-up energy.

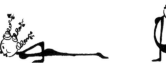

How to do it with style!

1 Lie on your stomach.

2 Bend your elbows and place your palms by your sides (just below the breast).

3 Leading with your chest and the crown of your head, lift your upper body off the floor.

4 Press your hands down firmly. Lift your chest to the ceiling, and bring your hips forward.

5 Lift your hips off the floor, keeping your thighs strong.

6 Bring your shoulder blades together and open up your chest.

7 Release your head back and look up.

HOLD FOR **5–15** SECONDS.

Other benefits

Great for relieving sciatic pain • Builds stamina • Strengthens arms and chest • Loosens stiff shoulders

Focus points

Keep your thighs strong and your knees lifted off the floor. Bring your shoulder blades in and open your chest.

ENERGY

BOOST & INVIGORATE

Forget the double espresso—coffee
provides only a short boost of energy,
while yoga boosts and sustains your
energy all day long!

Yoga recharges your creativity, invigorates
your mind, and gives you the energy you
need to get oodles of things done.

MEGA BENEFIT SEQUENCES

THE NUMBERS BELOW RESCUEGIRL CORRESPOND TO THE POSES.

SEQUENCE 1

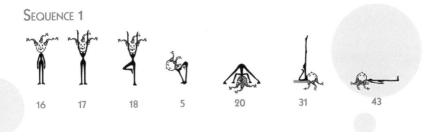

16   17   18   5   20   31   43

SEQUENCE 2

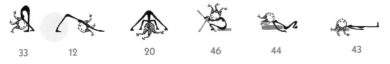

33   12   20   46   44   43

SEQUENCE 3

1   5   12   8   15   22   40   36   43

Tadasana
(mountain pose)

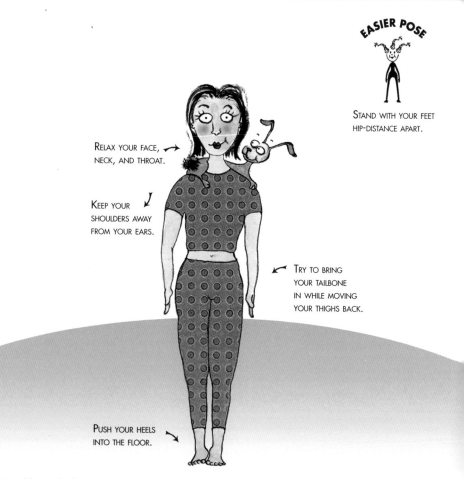

EASIER POSE

STAND WITH YOUR FEET
HIP-DISTANCE APART.

RELAX YOUR FACE,
NECK, AND THROAT.

KEEP YOUR
SHOULDERS AWAY
FROM YOUR EARS.

TRY TO BRING
YOUR TAILBONE
IN WHILE MOVING
YOUR THIGHS BACK.

PUSH YOUR HEELS
INTO THE FLOOR.

Lacking those bright eyes and bushy tail? This helps you perk up your energy.

How to do it with style!

1 Stand up straight with your feet together.

2 Spread your toes out like a fan.

3 Distribute your weight evenly across both feet.

4 Lift your kneecaps by tightening your thighs.

5 Move your thighs back and your tailbone in.

6 Straighten your arms with your palms facing in.

7 Pull your shoulder blades in and lift your chest.

8 Keep your neck and shoulders relaxed.

9 Look straight ahead.

HOLD FOR **1–2** MINUTES.

Other benefits

Strengthens and tones your whole body • Improves alignment • Creates balance

Focus points

Don't just stand passively! Activate every part of your body—from your heels to your head.

Urdhva Hastasana
(upward hand pose)

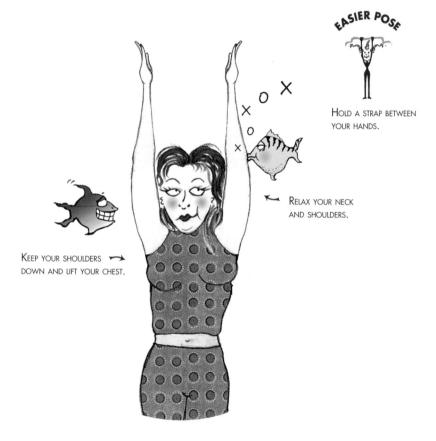

EASIER POSE

HOLD A STRAP BETWEEN YOUR HANDS.

RELAX YOUR NECK AND SHOULDERS.

KEEP YOUR SHOULDERS DOWN AND LIFT YOUR CHEST.

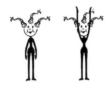

How to do it with style!

1 Stand with your feet hip-distance apart.

2 Lift your kneecaps by tightening your thighs.

3 Roll your shoulders back.

4 Extend your arms forward and lift them up.

5 Straighten your elbows, wrists, and fingers.

6 Relax your neck and shoulders.

7 Keep your head straight and look forward.

Other benefits

Alleviates stiff shoulders and arms • Releases tension in your upper back

Focus points

Activate your elbows and fingers and really open your chest.

HOLD FOR 30 SECONDS–1 MINUTE.
REPEAT 3 TIMES.

Vrksasana
(tree pose)

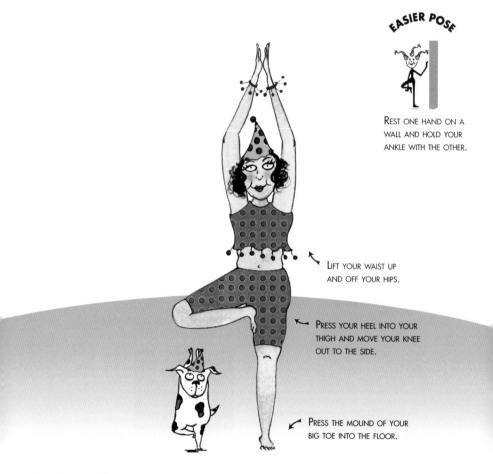

EASIER POSE

REST ONE HAND ON A WALL AND HOLD YOUR ANKLE WITH THE OTHER.

LIFT YOUR WAIST UP AND OFF YOUR HIPS.

PRESS YOUR HEEL INTO YOUR THIGH AND MOVE YOUR KNEE OUT TO THE SIDE.

PRESS THE MOUND OF YOUR BIG TOE INTO THE FLOOR.

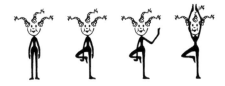

How to do it with style!

1 Stand with your feet together.

2 Bend your right knee and hold your ankle.

3 Place the heel of your right foot at the top of your left thigh.

4 Point your right knee out and your toes down.

5 Straighten your left leg as you press the right heel into your left thigh.

6 Stretch your arms overhead and press your palms together.

7 Look straight ahead.

HOLD FOR **30** SECONDS.
REPEAT ON THE OTHER SIDE.

Other benefits

Improves physical balance
• Calms your nerves •
Strengthens ankles, knees,
and hips

Focus points

Keep your hips even; don't
let one of them ride up.
Don't hyper-extend the knee
of your standing leg.

Dandasana
(staff pose)

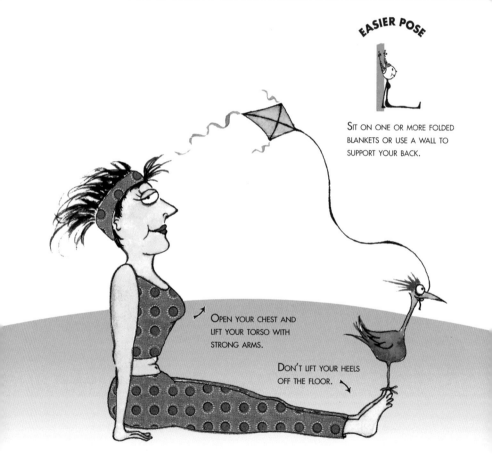

EASIER POSE

SIT ON ONE OR MORE FOLDED BLANKETS OR USE A WALL TO SUPPORT YOUR BACK.

OPEN YOUR CHEST AND LIFT YOUR TORSO WITH STRONG ARMS.

DON'T LIFT YOUR HEELS OFF THE FLOOR.

Need some wind beneath your wings?
This helps stimulate your respiratory system.

19
ENERGY

How to do it with style!

1 Sit on the floor with your feet stretched out in front of you.

2 Center yourself on your sitting bones.

3 Pull the bottom of your thigh away from your leg.

4 With your legs and feet together, press them firmly down into the floor.

5 Put your hands by your hips facing forward.

6 Pressing your hands down, lift your waist off your hips.

7 Roll your shoulders back and open your chest.

8 Relax your neck and shoulders.

HOLD FOR **30** SECONDS.
REPEAT **3** TIMES.

Other benefits

Stimulates the reproductive system • Relieves a stressed or tired back • Improves posture

Focus points

Engage every muscle in your legs and hips. Sit up tall—as if you are being pulled up by a string!

Prasarita Padottanasana
(extended leg intense stretch pose)

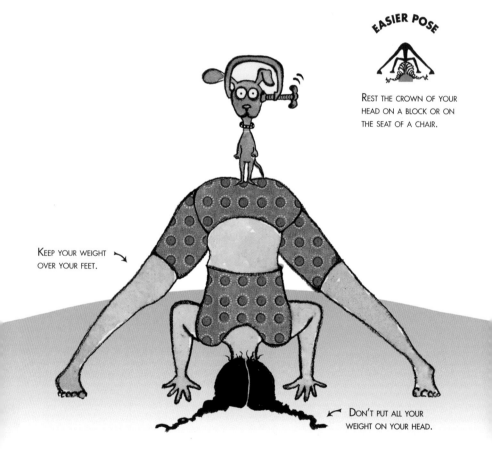

EASIER POSE

REST THE CROWN OF YOUR HEAD ON A BLOCK OR ON THE SEAT OF A CHAIR.

KEEP YOUR WEIGHT OVER YOUR FEET.

DON'T PUT ALL YOUR WEIGHT ON YOUR HEAD.

Feel like your head is in a vise?
This relieves a tension headache.

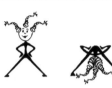

How to do it with style!

1 Stand with your legs a comfortable width apart.

2 Put your hands on your hips.

3 Stretch your torso forward and put your hands on the floor.

4 Lift your kneecaps by tightening your thighs.

5 Keep your legs straight and move your thighs back.

6 Place the crown of your head on the floor.

7 Press your palms into the floor.

HOLD FOR **30** SECONDS–**1** MINUTE.

Other benefits

Calms the brain • Strengthens the legs and spine • Tones your abdominal organs

Focus points

Keep your weight over your legs; don't lean forward onto your head. Keep your arms parallel to each other.

Virabhadrasana III
(warrior pose 3)

EASIER POSE

PLACE YOUR HANDS ON
THE BACK OF A CHAIR.

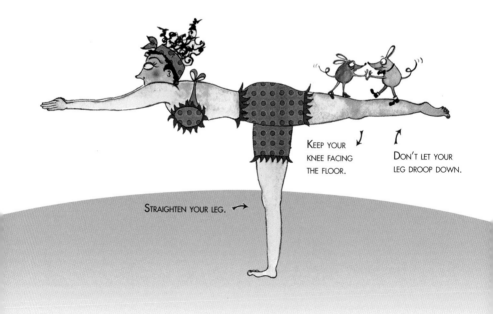

KEEP YOUR
KNEE FACING
THE FLOOR.

DON'T LET YOUR
LEG DROOP DOWN.

STRAIGHTEN YOUR LEG.

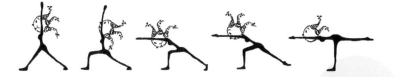

How to do it with style!

1 Stand with your right foot forward.

2 Your torso should also face forward.

3 Raise your arms straight over your head.

4 Bend your right knee, and extend your torso forward.

5 As you straighten your right leg, lift your left leg.

6 Stretch your arms ahead and shift your weight forward.

7 Look down at the floor for balance.

8 Your arms and lifted leg should form a line.

9 Lift your head and gaze past your hands.

HOLD FOR **30** SECONDS.
REPEAT ON THE OTHER SIDE.

Other benefits

Improves balance, memory, and concentration • Tones the entire body

Focus points

Open up your chest. Keep your bent knee over your heel. Lift your torso up off your hips and lean back slightly.

Dhanurasana
(bow pose)

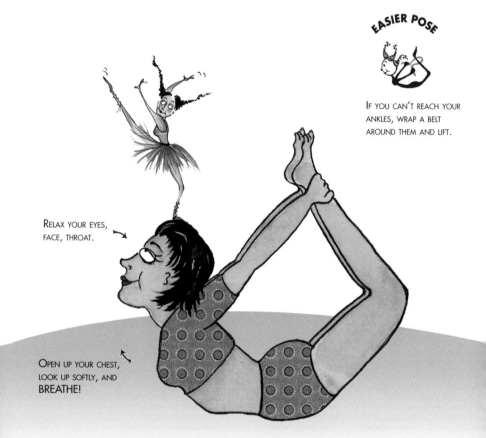

EASIER POSE

If you can't reach your ankles, wrap a belt around them and lift.

Relax your eyes, face, throat.

Open up your chest, look up softly, and BREATHE!

Feel like a rusty old nail?
This helps loosen joints and improves
your mobility.

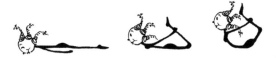

How to do it with style!

1 Lie on your tummy with your forehead on the floor.

2 Bend your knees and bring your feet toward your hips.

3 Hold your ankles with both hands.

4 Tighten your rear end and lift your chest, knees, and thighs up off the floor.

5 Both your ribs and thighs should be off the floor.

6 Center your weight on your belly button.

HOLD FOR **5–10** SECONDS.

Other benefits

Rejuvenates your spine •
Relieves an upset stomach
and constipation •
Strengthens your back

Focus points

Having an even arc from
your head to your toes is
more important than how
high you can lift your torso
and legs off the floor.

RESTORE

FEEL LIKE A KID AGAIN

True beauty isn't a wrinkle-free smile.
True beauty comes from within, but let's be
honest, we all want to look
and feel gorgeous...

Yoga slows the aging process by reducing
stress hormones, firming up the skin,
and creating more flexiblity...making you
radiantly beautiful inside *and* out!

MEGA BENEFIT SEQUENCES

THE NUMBERS BELOW RESCUEGIRL CORRESPOND
TO THE POSES.

SEQUENCE 1

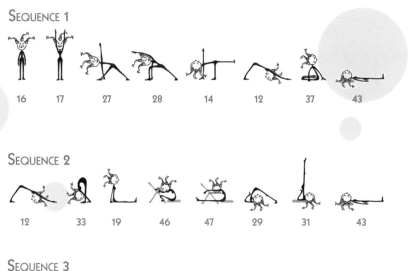

16   17   27   28   14   12   37   43

SEQUENCE 2

12   33   19   46   47   29   31   43

SEQUENCE 3

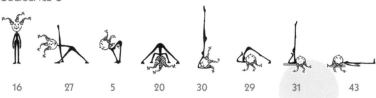

16   27   5   20   30   29   31   43

Paschima Namaskarasana
(back body prayer pose)

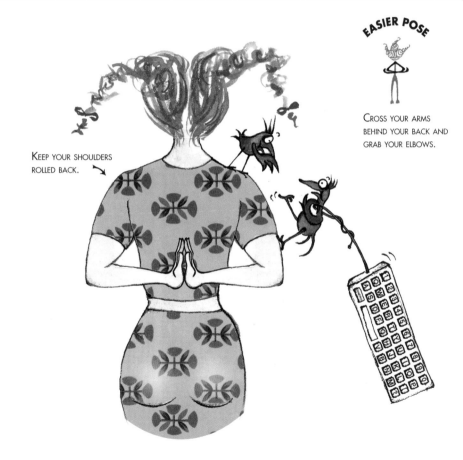

EASIER POSE

CROSS YOUR ARMS BEHIND YOUR BACK AND GRAB YOUR ELBOWS.

KEEP YOUR SHOULDERS ROLLED BACK.

Slave to the keyboard? This invigorates your hands, wrists, and shoulders.

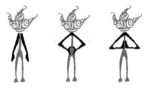

How to do it with style!

1 Roll your shoulders back and lift your chest.

2 Press your fingertips together behind your back.

3 Rotate your arms and wrists inward until your fingers point up to the sky (palms together).

4 Slide your hands up your back until they rest between your shoulder blades.

5 Press your palms firmly together.

HOLD FOR 30 SECONDS–1 MINUTE.

Other benefits

Straightens drooping shoulders • Strengthens wrists • Soothes upper back

Focus points

Keep even pressure on both your hands and press them firmly together.

Virasana
(hero pose)

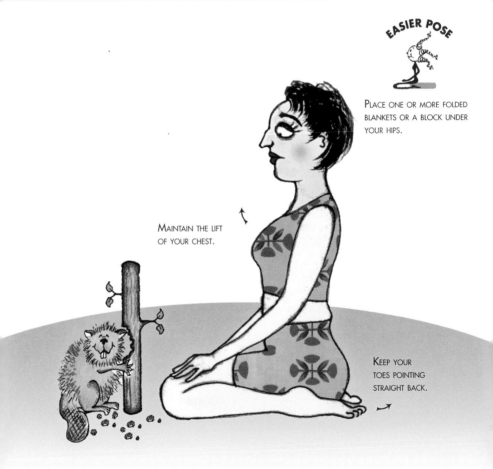

EASIER POSE

PLACE ONE OR MORE FOLDED BLANKETS OR A BLOCK UNDER YOUR HIPS.

MAINTAIN THE LIFT OF YOUR CHEST.

KEEP YOUR TOES POINTING STRAIGHT BACK.

Do your knees feel worn down?
This helps soothe and strengthen them.

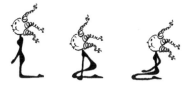

How to do it with style!

1 Kneel on the floor with your knees together and your feet wider apart than your hips.

2 Point your toes straight back.

3 Wedge your fingers into the back of your knees and draw your calf muscles outward and toward your heels, so you're not sitting on your calf muscles.

4 Center yourself on your sit bones.

5 Your heels should touch the sides of your hips.

6 Pull your shoulder blades back and lift your chest.

7 Rest your hands on your thighs.

HOLD FOR **30** SECONDS–**3** MINUTES.

Other benefits

Improves circulation to the pelvis • Deeply stretches muscles in the lower body

Focus points

Pretend bricks are on your thighs pressing them and your butt into the floor. Lift your torso to the sky.

Paschimottanasana
(intense stretch of the west pose)

PLACE ONE OR MORE FOLDED BLANKETS UNDER YOUR DERRIERE. WRAP A BELT AROUND YOUR FEET AND LEAN FORWARD.

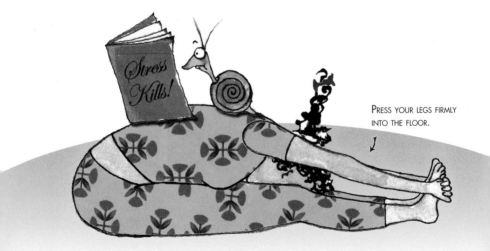

Stress Kills!

PRESS YOUR LEGS FIRMLY INTO THE FLOOR.

How to do it with style!

1 Sit with your legs stretched out in front of you.

2 Lift your chest and torso.

3 Raise your arms over your head.

4 Exhale and bend forward, leading with your chest.

5 Hold the sides of your feet and gently pull forward.

6 Lower your torso onto your legs, taking your chin to your shins.

HOLD FOR **20–30** SECONDS.

Other benefits

Reduces anxiety • Quiets your mind • Relaxes back muscles

Focus points

Don't let your butt come up off the floor. Allow your spine to stretch with each breath.

Supta Padangusthasana I
(reclined big toe pose 1)

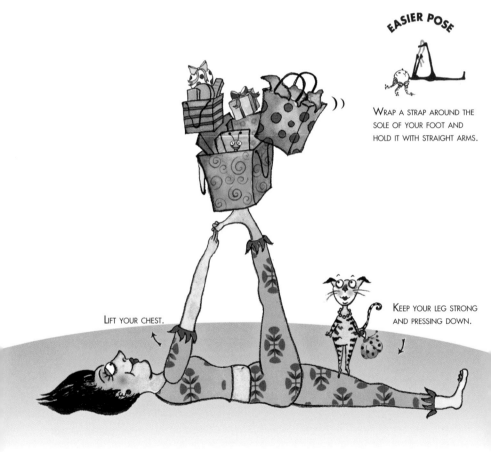

EASIER POSE

WRAP A STRAP AROUND THE SOLE OF YOUR FOOT AND HOLD IT WITH STRAIGHT ARMS.

LIFT YOUR CHEST.

KEEP YOUR LEG STRONG AND PRESSING DOWN.

Shopped 'til you dropped?
This pose soothes a sore back.

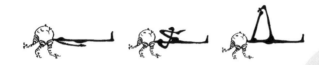

How to do it with style!

1 Lie down on the floor.

2 Bring your right knee to your chest.

3 Hold the big toe with the first two fingers of your right hand.

4 Straighten your right leg vertically.

5 Keep both legs straight and strong.

HOLD FOR **30** SECONDS.
REPEAT ON THE OTHER SIDE.

Other benefits

Relaxes hip joints • Eases menstrual pain • Tones the spine • Eases a stiff lower back and the back of your legs

Focus points

Actively press your leg and hips into the floor; don't let them ride up.

Utthita Trikonasana
(extended triangle pose)

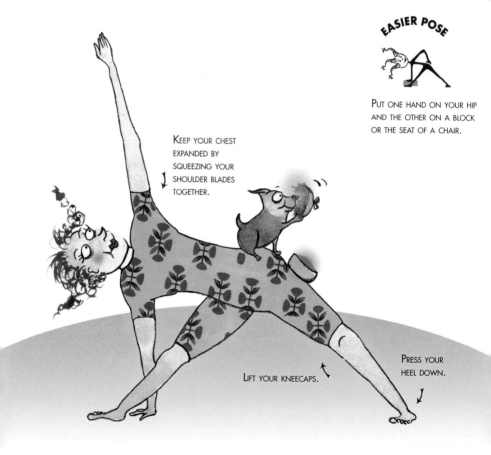

EASIER POSE

PUT ONE HAND ON YOUR HIP AND THE OTHER ON A BLOCK OR THE SEAT OF A CHAIR.

KEEP YOUR CHEST EXPANDED BY SQUEEZING YOUR SHOULDER BLADES TOGETHER.

LIFT YOUR KNEECAPS.

PRESS YOUR HEEL DOWN.

Looking a bit pale?
This gives your cheeks a rosy glow.

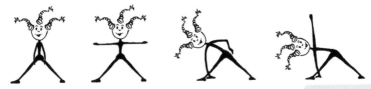

How to do it with style!

1 Stand with your legs a comfortable width apart.

2 Raise your arms to shoulder height.

3 Turn your right foot out 90° and turn your left toes slightly in. Align your heels.

4 Extend and bend your torso to the right, and place your right hand on the floor behind your right foot.

5 Reach up with your left hand, keeping your arm in line with your shoulder.

6 Turn your head and look up at your left thumb.

HOLD FOR **15** SECONDS.
REPEAT ON THE OTHER SIDE.

Other benefits

Tones legs—especially hamstrings • Improves posture • Strengthens pelvic region

Focus points

Anchor your legs and keep them strong.

Utthita Parsvakonasana
(extended side angle pose)

EASIER POSE

PUT YOUR BOTTOM HAND
ON A BLOCK AND YOUR
TOP HAND ON YOUR HIP.

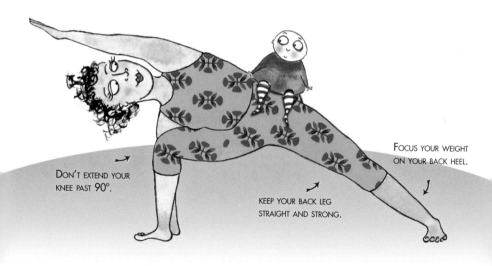

DON'T EXTEND YOUR
KNEE PAST 90°.

KEEP YOUR BACK LEG
STRAIGHT AND STRONG.

FOCUS YOUR WEIGHT
ON YOUR BACK HEEL.

Is baby glued to your hip all day?
This helps relieve sciatica and a tired back.

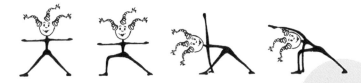

How to do it with style!

1 Stand with your legs a comfortable width apart.

2 Raise your arms to shoulder height.

3 Turn your right foot out 90° and bring your left toes slightly in. Align your heels.

4 Bend your right leg at the knee until your thigh is parallel to the floor.

5 Place your right hand on the floor behind your right foot.

6 Stretch the left arm over your left ear.

7 Turn your head and look up at the extended arm.

8 Move your chest up and back, so your hips and legs are in a line.

HOLD FOR **20–30** SECONDS.
REPEAT ON THE OTHER SIDE.

Other benefits

Strengthens legs • Improves circulation in your feet • Helps relieve gas and indigestion

Focus points

Make sure your chest does not tilt toward the floor; it should remain perpendicular to the floor.

Halasana
(plough pose)

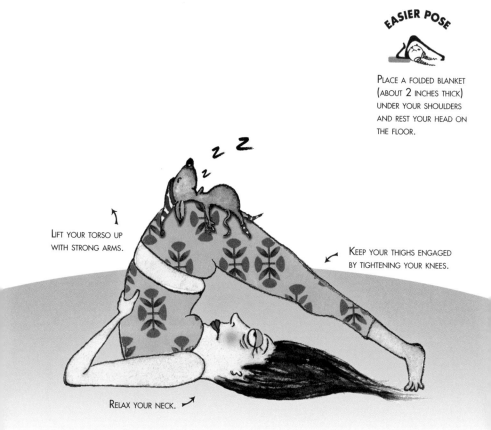

EASIER POSE

PLACE A FOLDED BLANKET (ABOUT 2 INCHES THICK) UNDER YOUR SHOULDERS AND REST YOUR HEAD ON THE FLOOR.

LIFT YOUR TORSO UP WITH STRONG ARMS.

KEEP YOUR THIGHS ENGAGED BY TIGHTENING YOUR KNEES.

RELAX YOUR NECK.

Too familiar with late-night TV?
This helps reduce insomnia.

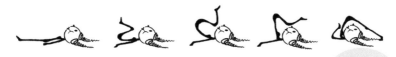

How to do it with style!

1 Lie on your back with your arms at your sides.

2 Roll your shoulders under and away from your ears.

3 Bend your knees and bring them to your chest.

4 Press down with your hands and swing your legs up and over your head.

5 Place your toes on the floor behind you.

6 Put your palms on your torso for support and push your back up toward the sky.

7 Lift your tailbone toward the sky. Keep your legs straight.

HOLD FOR 1–3 MINUTES.

Other benefits

Lifts your spirits • Relaxes your mind • Stretches your shoulders and spine • Reduces fatigue

Focus points

Keep your torso perpendicular to the floor and your legs fully extended. Move your chin away from your chest and soften your neck.

Salamba Sirsasana
(headstand pose)

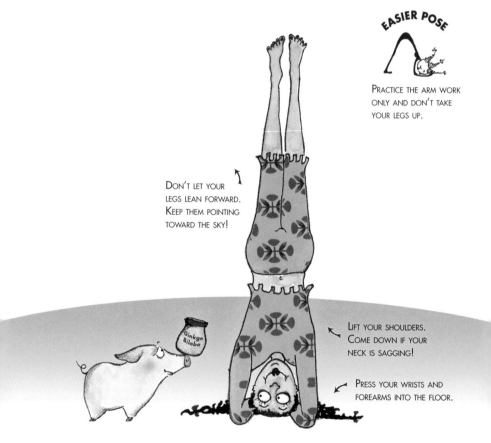

EASIER POSE

PRACTICE THE ARM WORK ONLY AND DON'T TAKE YOUR LEGS UP.

DON'T LET YOUR LEGS LEAN FORWARD. KEEP THEM POINTING TOWARD THE SKY!

Ginkgo Biloba

LIFT YOUR SHOULDERS. COME DOWN IF YOUR NECK IS SAGGING!

PRESS YOUR WRISTS AND FOREARMS INTO THE FLOOR.

How to do it with style!

1 Kneel on the floor in front of a wall.

2 Interlock your fingers and open your palms.

3 Place your knuckles at the wall and your elbows shoulder-width apart.

4 Press your forearms into the floor.

5 Place the crown of your head on the floor just in front of your cupped hands.

6 Slide your head into your palms.

7 Press your wrists into the floor.

8 Lift your shoulders away from your ears.

9 Straighten and lift your legs up to the wall (one at a time if necessary).

HOLD FOR 5-10 SECONDS.

Other benefits

Energizes the body •
Improves circulation •
Stimulates your nervous
system • Tones neck
muscles

Focus points

Keep your weight evenly
balanced on your forearms.
Lift your tailbone toward
your heels. Keep your legs
long and straight.

Salamba Sarvangasana
(shoulder stand pose)

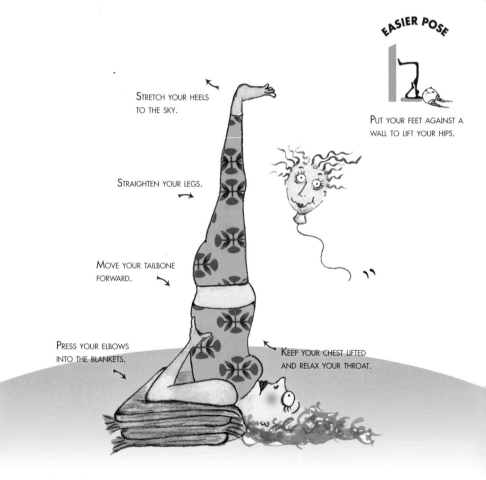

EASIER POSE

PUT YOUR FEET AGAINST A
WALL TO LIFT YOUR HIPS.

STRETCH YOUR HEELS
TO THE SKY.

STRAIGHTEN YOUR LEGS.

MOVE YOUR TAILBONE
FORWARD.

PRESS YOUR ELBOWS
INTO THE BLANKETS.

KEEP YOUR CHEST LIFTED
AND RELAX YOUR THROAT.

Feel like you've lost your head?
This soothes those frazzled nerves.

How to do it with style!

1 Lie on folded blankets with your shoulders supported and your head on the floor.

2 With your arms at your sides, bring your knees to your chest.

3 Press down with your hands and lift your hips over your shoulders, so your torso is perpendicular to the floor.

4 Lift your hips and torso straight up, supporting the middle of your back with your hands.

5 Keep your elbows close together.

6 Lift your chest to your chin.

7 Straighten your legs.

HOLD FOR 30 SECONDS.

Other benefits

Tones organs • Stretches shoulders and neck • Improves digestion

Focus points

Press the back of your upper arms and your shoulders into the blankets. Lift your upper spine away from the floor.

CLEANSE

Detox & Purify

What would life be without blinis
and bad habits?

Thank goodness yoga has the power to
restore, repair, and replenish! It boosts
the circulation of blood and lymph fluid,
strengthens the endocrine system, and
flushes toxins out of your body.

MEGA BENEFIT SEQUENCES

THE NUMBERS BELOW RESCUEGIRL CORRESPOND
TO THE POSES.

SEQUENCE 1

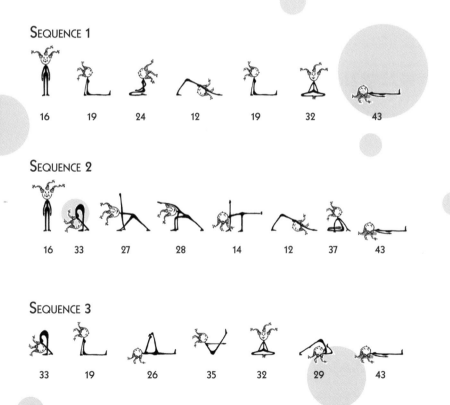

16   19   24   12   19   32   43

SEQUENCE 2

16   33   27   28   14   12   37   43

SEQUENCE 3

33   19   26   35   32   29   43

Baddhakonasana
(bound angle pose)

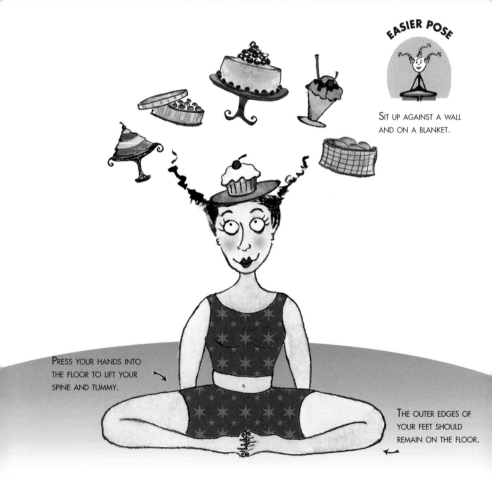

EASIER POSE

SIT UP AGAINST A WALL
AND ON A BLANKET.

PRESS YOUR HANDS INTO
THE FLOOR TO LIFT YOUR
SPINE AND TUMMY.

THE OUTER EDGES OF
YOUR FEET SHOULD
REMAIN ON THE FLOOR.

Eating everything but the kitchen sink?
This helps relieve a stuffed tummy.

How to do it with style!

1 Sit with your legs in front of you.

2 Bend one leg at a time and place the soles of your feet together.

3 Bring your heels close to your body.

4 Push your knees down toward the floor.

5 Use your thumbs to open the inner edges of your feet like a book.

6 Bring your shoulder blades together and open up your chest.

7 Press your fingertips down on the floor behind you.

HOLD FOR **1–5** MINUTES.

Other benefits

Increases hip and leg flexibility • Strengthens bladder and uterus • Alleviates tension in your back • Eases menstrual cramps and heavy bleeding

Focus points

Press your knees, ankles, and thighs down and stretch your torso upward. Hold your feet firmly together to really lift the torso.

Uttanasana
(intense forward stretch pose)

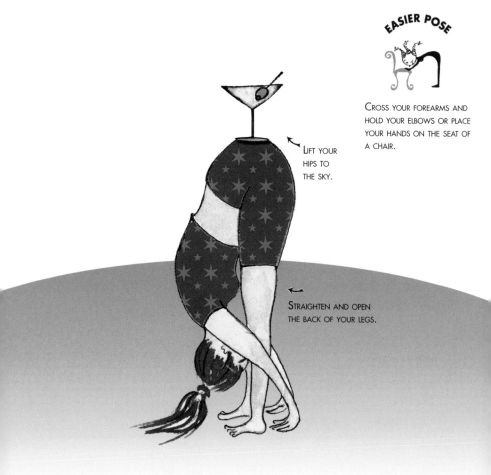

EASIER POSE

CROSS YOUR FOREARMS AND HOLD YOUR ELBOWS OR PLACE YOUR HANDS ON THE SEAT OF A CHAIR.

LIFT YOUR HIPS TO THE SKY.

STRAIGHTEN AND OPEN THE BACK OF YOUR LEGS.

Does every bartender in town know you? This soothes a hangover.

How to do it with style!

1 Stand with your feet hip-distance apart.

2 Lift your kneecaps to tighten your thighs.

3 Bend forward from your hips.

4 Lift your waist and move your chest forward.

5 Bring your torso toward your thighs.

6 With your knees straight, bring your palms behind your ankles.

7 Press your heels firmly into the floor and lift your butt toward the ceiling.

8 Let your head hang down.

HOLD FOR **30** SECONDS–**1** MINUTE.

Other benefits

Stimulates liver and kidneys • Relieves headache and insomnia • Reduces fatigue and anxiety

Focus points

With each exhalation move more fully into the bend. Keep your legs strong and straight.

Marichyasana I
(Marichi's pose 1)

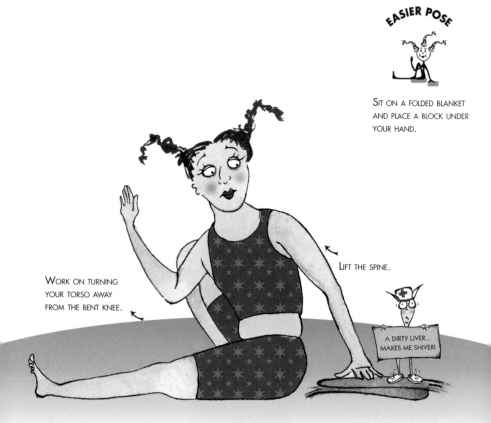

EASIER POSE

SIT ON A FOLDED BLANKET AND PLACE A BLOCK UNDER YOUR HAND.

LIFT THE SPINE.

WORK ON TURNING YOUR TORSO AWAY FROM THE BENT KNEE.

A DIRTY LIVER... MAKES ME SHIVER!

Would you be rejected as an organ donor?
This tones and detoxifies organs.

How to do it with style!

1 Sit with your legs stretched out in front of you.

2 Bend your right leg and pull your heel toward your sitting bone. Keep your foot flat on the floor.

3 Keep the left leg stretched and strong.

4 Place your left fingertips behind you.

5 Bend your right elbow, and place the upper arm against the inside of your right thigh.

6 Press your right arm and knee against each other.

7 Lift your torso and twist to the left.

HOLD FOR 30 SECONDS–1 MINUTE.
REPEAT ON THE OTHER SIDE.

Other benefits

Rejuvenates and tones the liver, kidney, and spleen • Releases tension in your neck, shoulders, and back

Focus points

Keep your straight leg and the foot of the bent-knee leg grounded. Twist a little more with each exhalation.

Paripurna Navasana
(full boat pose)

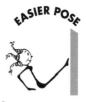

EASIER POSE

PLACE YOUR HEELS ON A
WALL AND YOUR HANDS ON
THE FLOOR BEHIND YOUR HIPS.

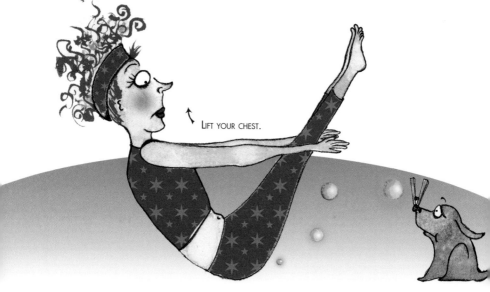

LIFT YOUR CHEST.

Are you full of beans?
This helps eliminate gas and bloating.

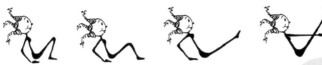

How to do it with style!

1 Sit on the floor with your knees bent.

2 Put your hands at your sides a little bit behind your hips (fingers facing forward).

3 Lean your torso back as you raise your feet off the floor and straighten your legs; don't round your back.

4 Straighten your knees and raise the tips of your toes slightly above eye level.

5 Stretch your arms alongside your legs and parallel to the floor with your palms facing each other.

6 Roll your shoulders back and lift your chest.

HOLD FOR 10–20 SECONDS.

Other benefits

Strengthens abdominals, hip flexors, and spine • Improves digestion • Stimulates intestines, kidneys, and thyroid

Focus points

Weight should be balanced between your sitting bones and your tailbone. Open your chest and don't round your back.

Bharadvajasana
(Bharadvaja's pose)

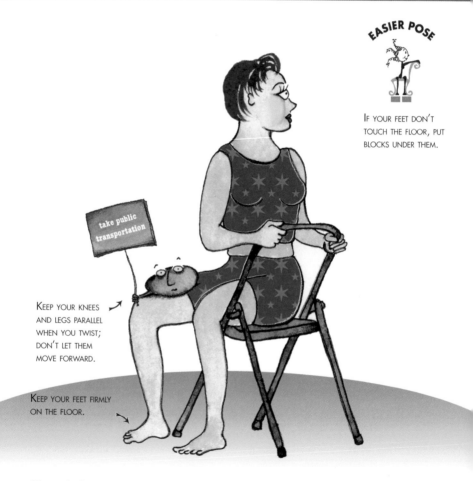

EASIER POSE

IF YOUR FEET DON'T
TOUCH THE FLOOR, PUT
BLOCKS UNDER THEM.

take public
transportation

KEEP YOUR KNEES
AND LEGS PARALLEL
WHEN YOU TWIST;
DON'T LET THEM
MOVE FORWARD.

KEEP YOUR FEET FIRMLY
ON THE FLOOR.

Spending too much time behind the wheel? This refreshes the spine.

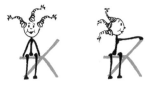

How to do it with style!

1 Sit sideways on a chair with your thighs supported.

2 Place your feet hip-distance apart directly under your knees.

3 Lift your waist off your hips and open your chest.

4 Hold on to the sides of the chair back. Lift your elbows up and out to the sides.

5 Pull the chair toward you with the close hand and push the chair away from you with your far hand.

6 Twist a little more with each exhalation.

7 Look over your left shoulder.

HOLD FOR **30** SECONDS–**1** MINUTE.
REPEAT ON THE OTHER SIDE.

Other benefits

Stretches spine, shoulders, and hips • Relieves lower-back ache, neck pain, and sciatica

Focus points

Keep your butt and your hips cemented to the chair. Don't turn or lift your hips when you twist—focus on twisting your torso only.

Bharadvajasana I
(Bharadvaja's pose 1)

EASIER POSE

PLACE A FOLDED BLANKET UNDER THE SIT BONE YOU'RE TURNING TOWARD AND PLACE A BLOCK UNDER THE HAND BEHIND YOU.

DON'T LET YOUR BACK THIGH OR HIP COME UP OFF THE FLOOR AS YOU TWIST.

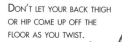

Could you be King Tut's sister?
This pose enlivens and refreshes.

37
CLEANSE

How to do it with style!

1 Sit with your legs stretched out in front of you.

2 Bend your knees and bring both feet to the right side at your hip. Your knees are facing forward.

3 Place your right ankle over the arch of your left foot.

4 Place your right hand over your left thigh.

5 Put your left fingers on the floor behind your right hip.

6 Press the right shoulder blade into your back.

7 Lift your waist up off your hips and twist to the left.

8 Turn your head to look past your shoulder.

HOLD FOR **30** SECONDS–**1** MINUTE.
REPEAT ON THE OTHER SIDE.

Other benefits

Massages reproductive organs • Energizes adrenal glands • Improves spine and hip flexibility

Focus points

Lift your torso a little with every inhalation—push your fingers into the floor to help. With every exhalation twist a little more.

SANITY

MOOD & BALANCE

Who needs Prozac® when
you've got pranayama*?

Goodies like an overall sense of
well-being and mental equilibrium are
just two of the benefits that regular
yoga practice brings you.

*Pranayama = life force or vital energy that
permeates the universe at all levels.

MEGA BENEFIT SEQUENCES

THE NUMBERS BELOW RescueGirl CORRESPOND
TO THE POSES.

SEQUENCE 1

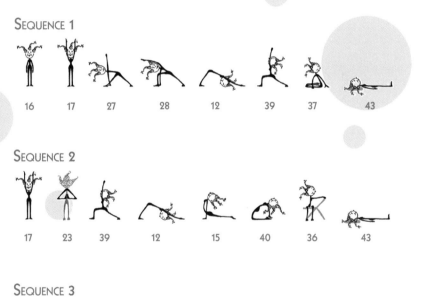

16   17   27   28   12   39   37   43

SEQUENCE 2

17   23   39   12   15   40   36   43

SEQUENCE 3

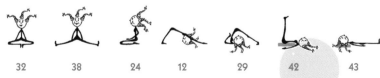

32   38   24   12   29   42   43

Upavistha Konasana
(seated wide angle pose)

EASIER POSE

Sᴉᴛ ᴏɴ ᴀ ꜰᴏʟᴅᴇᴅ ʙʟᴀɴᴋᴇᴛ.

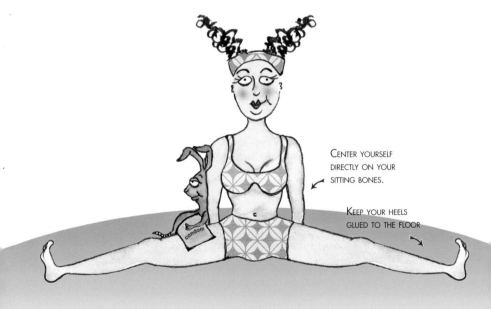

Cᴇɴᴛᴇʀ ʏᴏᴜʀsᴇʟꜰ
ᴅɪʀᴇᴄᴛʟʏ ᴏɴ ʏᴏᴜʀ
sɪᴛᴛɪɴɢ ʙᴏɴᴇs.

Kᴇᴇᴘ ʏᴏᴜʀ ʜᴇᴇʟs
ɢʟᴜᴇᴅ ᴛᴏ ᴛʜᴇ ꜰʟᴏᴏʀ

Lost your libido?
This finds it in an instant.

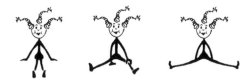

How to do it with style!

1 Sit with your legs stretched out in front of you.

2 Move each leg out to the side, one at a time, forming a 90° angle.

3 Your knees and toes should point straight up.

4 Place your hands behind you at your hips.

5 Press your hands against the floor and slide your hips forward, widening your legs another 10° or so.

6 Press down with your legs so they are flat on the floor.

7 Roll your shoulders back and lift your chest.

HOLD FOR 1-3 MINUTES.

Other benefits

Increases circulation to the pelvic area • Stimulates ovaries • Lifts and tones uterus • Relaxes the groin area

Focus points

Sit up tall. Actively press your legs into the floor and lift your torso.

Virabhadrasana I
(warrior pose 1)

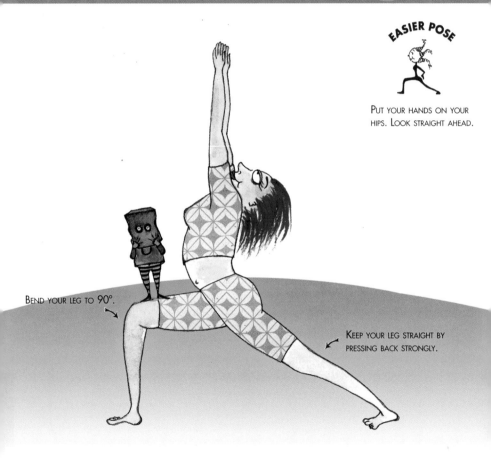

EASIER POSE

PUT YOUR HANDS ON YOUR
HIPS. LOOK STRAIGHT AHEAD.

BEND YOUR LEG TO 90°.

KEEP YOUR LEG STRAIGHT BY
PRESSING BACK STRONGLY.

Feel like hiding?
This increases your self-confidence.

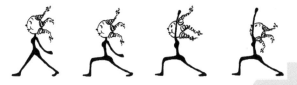

How to do it with style!

1 Step your right foot forward until your legs are wide apart. Keep your feet hip-distance apart.

2 Turn your right foot in slightly and your left foot out to 90°.

3 Lift your waist up and off your hips.

4 Slide your knee forward until it is directly over your ankle—no further.

5 Lift your arms straight up over your head, palms facing together and elbows straight.

6 Drop your shoulders down and back.

7 Carefully arch your back and look up to the sky.

HOLD FOR **30** SECONDS–**1** MINUTE.
REPEAT ON THE OTHER SIDE.

Other benefits

Improves concentration and balance • Relieves joint stiffness • Improves breathing and circulation

Focus points

Keep your arms and upper torso lifting strongly toward the sky while your legs and lower torso drop down to the floor.

Ustrasana
(camel pose)

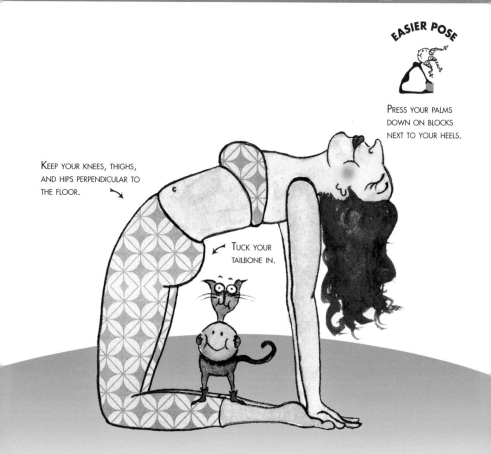

EASIER POSE

PRESS YOUR PALMS DOWN ON BLOCKS NEXT TO YOUR HEELS.

KEEP YOUR KNEES, THIGHS, AND HIPS PERPENDICULAR TO THE FLOOR.

TUCK YOUR TAILBONE IN.

Feel like you're going to cloud up and rain?
This lifts your spirits.

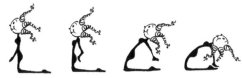

How to do it with style!

1 Kneel with your legs hip-distance apart. Point your toes straight back.

2 Place your hands on your hips and tuck your tailbone in.

3 Keep your chest lifted and pull your elbows straight back.

4 Reach for your feet and press your palms down on your heels.

5 Squeeze your shoulder blades together and lift your chest.

6 Release your head back.

HOLD FOR **30** SECONDS–**1** MINUTE.

Other benefits

Increases lung capacity • Strengthens spine and upper back • Improves posture

Focus points

Be careful not to strain your neck. Keep your throat relaxed. Don't forget to breathe!

Urdhva Dhanurasana
(upward facing bow pose)

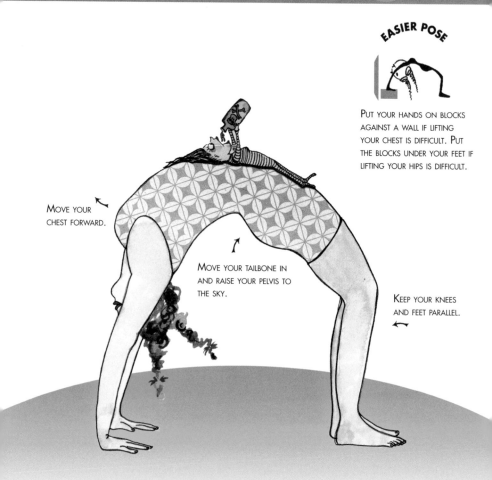

EASIER POSE

PUT YOUR HANDS ON BLOCKS AGAINST A WALL IF LIFTING YOUR CHEST IS DIFFICULT. PUT THE BLOCKS UNDER YOUR FEET IF LIFTING YOUR HIPS IS DIFFICULT.

MOVE YOUR CHEST FORWARD.

MOVE YOUR TAILBONE IN AND RAISE YOUR PELVIS TO THE SKY.

KEEP YOUR KNEES AND FEET PARALLEL.

Feeling a bit blue? This turns your mood a lovely shade of pink.

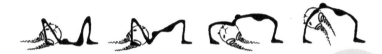

How to do it with style!

1 Lie on your back.

2 Bend your knees and rest your heels near your butt.

3 Place your palms on either side of your head, your fingers pointing toward your feet.

4 Press your palms and feet firmly into the floor.

5 Exhale and lift your chest and butt off the floor.

6 Place the top of your head on the floor.

7 Pause.

8 Pressing up with your arms and legs, lift your head off the floor and bring your body into an arch.

9 Release your head down.

HOLD FOR **5–10** SECONDS.

Other benefits

Energizes the nervous system • Increases flexibility of the spine and chest • Boosts overall energy

Focus points

Keep the front of your body relaxed and the back of your body strong. Keep your tummy muscles passive so you can breathe easily.

Viparita Karani
(inverted lake pose)

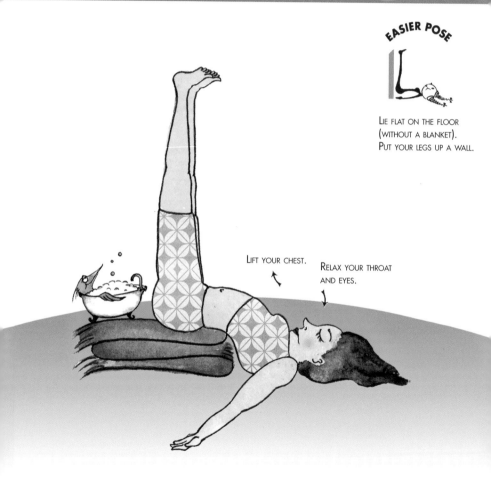

EASIER POSE

LIE FLAT ON THE FLOOR (WITHOUT A BLANKET). PUT YOUR LEGS UP A WALL.

LIFT YOUR CHEST.

RELAX YOUR THROAT AND EYES.

Beyond exhausted?
This rejuvenates the body.

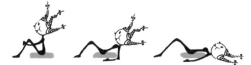

How to do it with style!

1 Sit on folded blankets.

2 Lie down with your head, shoulders, and upper back resting on the floor (your lower and middle back are on the blankets).

3 Slowly lift your legs, one at a time, until they are straight and in line with your hips.

4 Keep your spine arched by lifting your chest to your chin and resting your lower spine and hips on the blankets.

5 Spread your shoulder blades and release your arms and hands to your sides, palms up.

HOLD FOR **5–15** MINUTES.

Other benefits

Balances the endocrine system • Calms nerves • Relieves cramped legs

Focus points

Keep your legs firm enough to hold your thighs vertically. Let the weight of your tummy sink deeply into your torso.

Savasana
(corpse pose)

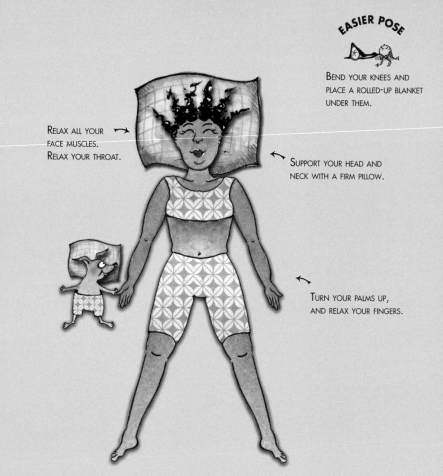

EASIER POSE

BEND YOUR KNEES AND PLACE A ROLLED-UP BLANKET UNDER THEM.

RELAX ALL YOUR FACE MUSCLES. RELAX YOUR THROAT.

SUPPORT YOUR HEAD AND NECK WITH A FIRM PILLOW.

TURN YOUR PALMS UP, AND RELAX YOUR FINGERS.

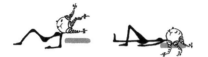

How to do it with style!

1 Sit on the floor with your knees bent and your feet on the floor. Lean back on your forearms.

2 Slowly extend your right leg, then your left, pushing through your heels.

3 Release both legs, letting your feet drop to the sides.

4 Lie back, resting on the back center of your skull.

5 Release your arms to the sides.

6 Turn your arms out, resting the back of your hands on the floor.

7 Let your eyes sink into the back of your head.

HOLD FOR 5-10 MINUTES.

Other benefits

Brings deep relaxation and serenity • Helps to lower blood pressure • Reduces headaches and fatigue

Focus points

Breathe slowly and deeply, letting a sense of calm relaxation envelop your whole body. Observe this loosening of your level of tension.

RAGTIME

PMS & Period Relief

Don't dread it, embrace it! What better excuse to pamper the lazy girl in you and welcome the opportunity to look inward?

Yoga will not only relieve the myriad symptoms that accompany your cycle, but will also clear your mind for self-exploration.

MEGA BENEFIT SEQUENCE

THE NUMBERS BELOW RESCUEGIRL CORRESPOND
TO THE POSES.

    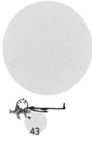

45 44 48 46 47 43

Supta Baddha Konasana
(reclining bound angle pose)

EASIER POSE

CROSS YOUR LEGS INSTEAD OF TOUCHING THE SOLES OF YOUR FEET TOGETHER.

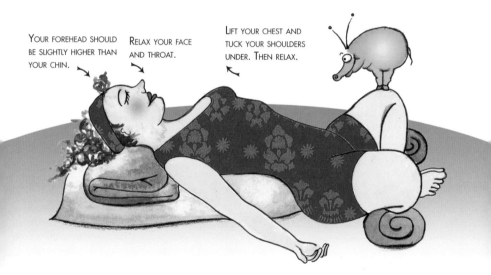

YOUR FOREHEAD SHOULD BE SLIGHTLY HIGHER THAN YOUR CHIN.

RELAX YOUR FACE AND THROAT.

LIFT YOUR CHEST AND TUCK YOUR SHOULDERS UNDER. THEN RELAX.

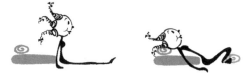

How to do it with style!

1 Place a bolster lengthwise behind your hips.

2 Put a rolled blanket on the far end.

3 Have two more rolled blankets within reach.

4 Stretch your legs out in front of you.

5 Bring the soles of your feet together.

6 Pull your heels close to your body.

7 Place a rolled blanket under each knee.

8 Lie back on your elbows.

9 Rest your torso evenly on the bolster.

10 Support your head and neck on the blanket.

11 Relax your arms at your sides, palms up.

HOLD FOR 5–10 MINUTES.

Other benefits

Relieves premenstrual and menstrual pain • Brings energy to reproductive organs • Loosens hips

Focus points

Relax completely. Let your face and jaw soften. Focus your attention inward.

Supta Virasana
(reclined hero's pose)

ADD HEIGHT TO THE
BOLSTER WITH BLANKETS TO
KEEP YOUR TORSO LIFTED.

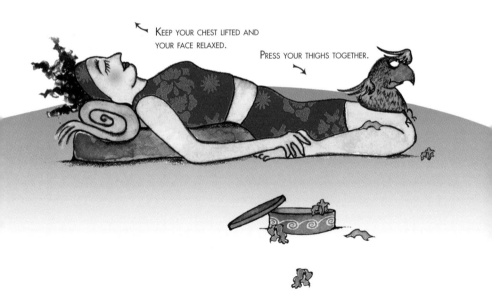

KEEP YOUR CHEST LIFTED AND
YOUR FACE RELAXED.

PRESS YOUR THIGHS TOGETHER.

Would you swap your beau for a
box of bonbons? This curbs your appetite.

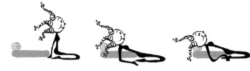

How to do it with style!

1 Place a bolster lengthwise behind your butt.

2 Put a rolled blanket on the far end of the bolster.

3 Kneel with your knees together in front of the bolster.

4 Spread your toes apart with the soles facing up.

5 Sit between your feet, centered on your sitting bones.

6 Lie back on your elbows.

7 Rest your torso evenly on the bolster.

8 Support your head and neck on the blanket.

HOLD FOR **1–5** MINUTES.

Other benefits

Relieves bloating, fullness, and indigestion • Relaxes thighs and groin • Rejuvenates tired legs

Focus points

Rest completely. Hold your toes and ankles close to your body, and point them straight back.

Adho Muhka Baddakonasana
(downward facing bound angle pose)

EASIER POSE

ADD MORE BLANKETS TO
THE CHAIR SEAT (OR LEAVE
YOUR HEAD UP IF YOUR
BACK IS STRAINED).

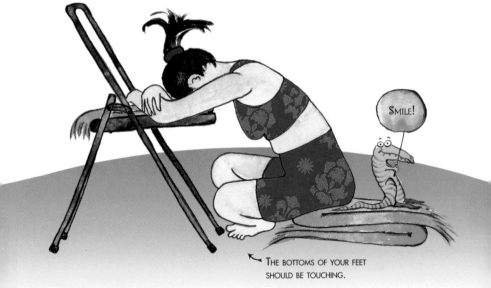

SMILE!

← THE BOTTOMS OF YOUR FEET
SHOULD BE TOUCHING.

Weepier than spring showers?
This helps alleviate hormonal tears.

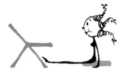

How to do it with style!

1 Sit in front of a chair on several folded blankets.

2 Place a folded blanket on the chair seat.

3 Bend your knees, one at a time, placing the soles of your feet together.

4 Sit up tall and lift your waist off your hips.

5 Keep your torso lifted as you lean forward, and place your hands on the chair seat.

6 Fold your arms and rest your forehead on your forearms.

HOLD FOR **1-3** MINUTES.

Other benefits

Relieves migraines and stress headaches • Counteracts nausea • Soothes nerves

Focus points

Relax completely. Empty your mind of all tension and worry.

Paschimottanasana
(intense stretch pose)

EASIER POSE

ADD MORE BLANKETS TO
THE CHAIR SEAT (OR KEEP
YOUR HEAD UP IF YOUR
BACK IS STRAINED).

REST YOUR ARMS COMFORTABLY
ON A CHAIR. USE MORE
BLANKETS IF NEEDED.

Hanging on by a thread?
This helps get you grounded.

How to do it with style!

1 Sit on several folded blankets in front of a chair with your legs stretched out under the chair.

2 Place a folded blanket on the chair seat.

3 Sit up tall and lift your waist off your hips.

4 Keep your torso lifted as you lean forward.

5 Place your arms on the chair seat, letting your hands and wrists dangle over the edge.

6 Rest your forehead on the seat of the chair.

HOLD FOR **1-3** MINUTES.

Other benefits

Calms the mind • Relieves stress and mild depression • Relieves menstrual discomfort

Focus points

With each inhalation, lift and lengthen your torso. With each exhalation, release a little further into the forward bend.

Sukasana
(cross-legged pose)

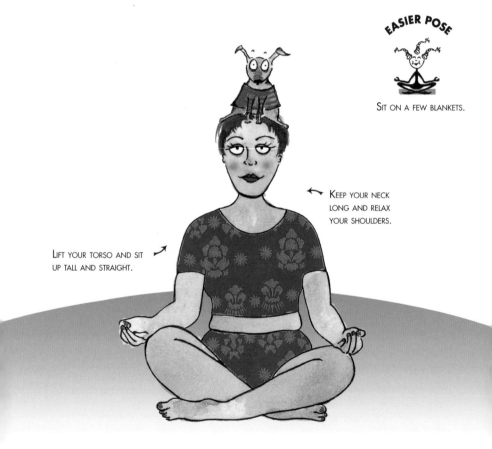

EASIER POSE

SIT ON A FEW BLANKETS.

KEEP YOUR NECK
LONG AND RELAX
YOUR SHOULDERS.

LIFT YOUR TORSO AND SIT
UP TALL AND STRAIGHT.

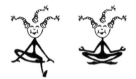

How to do it with style!

1 Sit with your legs stretched out in front of you.

2 Bend one leg and place your heel under the opposite thigh. Repeat with the other leg.

3 Sit up tall—spine, neck, and body erect.

4 Keep your abdomen strong and your head straight.

5 Place your hands on your knees, palms facing up.

6 Completely relax your body.

HOLD FOR **1–5** MINUTES.
REPEAT WITH LEGS CROSSED THE OPPOSITE WAY.

Other benefits

Creates inner harmony
• Raises awareness •
Rejuvenates tired legs
and back

Focus points

Keep your mind blank.
Mentally observe your
breath coming in and
going out.

POSES AT A GLANCE!

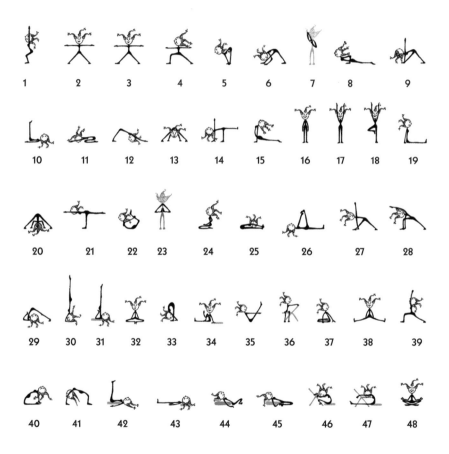

1   2   3   4   5   6   7   8   9

10   11   12   13   14   15   16   17   18   19

20   21   22   23   24   25   26   27   28

29   30   31   32   33   34   35   36   37   38   39

40   41   42   43   44   45   46   47   48

1. Utkatasana (chair pose)
2. Utthita Hasta Padasana (extended hand & foot pose)
3. Parsva Hasta Padasana (extended side hand & foot pose)
4. Virabhadrasana II (warrior pose 2)
5. Padangusthasana (foot & big toe pose)
6. Parsvottanasana (intense side stretch pose)
7. Gomukhasana (cow face pose—arms only)
8. Chaturanga Dandasana (four limb staff pose)
9. Parivrtta Trikonasana (revolving triangle pose)
10. Urdhva Prasarita Padasana (upward extended foot pose)
11. Adho Mukha Virasana (child's pose)
12. Adho Mukha Svanasana (downward facing dog pose)
13. Prasarita Padottanasana I (extended leg intense stretch pose 1)
14. Ardha Chandrasana (half moon pose)
15. Urdhva Mukha Svanasana (upward facing dog pose)
16. Tadasana (mountain pose)
17. Urdhva Hastasana (upward hand pose)
18. Vrksasana (tree pose)
19. Dandasana (staff pose)
20. Prasarita Padottanasana (extended leg intense stretch pose)
21. Virabhadrasana III (warrior pose 3)
22. Dhanurasana (bow pose)
23. Paschima Namaskarasana (back body prayer pose)
24. Virasana (hero pose)
25. Paschimottanasana (intense stretch of the west pose)

26. Supta Padangusthasana I (reclined big toe pose 1)
27. Utthita Trikonasana (extended triangle pose)
28. Utthita Parsvakonasana (extended side angle pose)
29. Halasana (plough pose)
30. Salamba Sirsasana (headstand pose)
31. Salamba Sarvangasana (shoulder stand pose)
32. Baddhakonasana (bound angle pose)
33. Uttanasana (intense forward stretch pose)
34. Marichyasana I (Marichi's pose 1)
35. Paripurna Navasana (full boat pose)
36. Bharadvajasana (Bharadvaja's pose)
37. Bharadvajasana I (Bharadvaja's pose 1)
38. Upavistha Konasana (seated wide angle pose)
39. Virabhadransana I (warrior pose 1)
40. Ustrasana (camel pose)
41. Urdhva Dhanurasana (upward facing bow pose)
42. Viparita Karani (inverted lake pose)
43. Savasana (corpse pose)
44. Supta Baddha Konasana (reclining bound angle pose)
45. Supta Virasana (reclined hero's pose)
46. Adho Mukha Baddakonasana (downward facing bound angle pose)
47. Paschimottanasana (intense stretch pose)
48. Sukasana (cross-legged pose)

A LITTLE YOGA EVERY DAY MAKES YOU SMILE AND KEEPS THE DOCTOR AWAY!

The Original RescueGirl

Writer/illustrator Amy Luwis has been inspired by the magical benefits of yoga for many years, so she researched like the dickens, interviewed yoga instructors, and put her friends in these poses. The result? This perfect little yoga book.

When Amy isn't doing her favorite pose (corpse pose) or doodling, she's busy with the nonprofit organization she co-founded, 1-800-Save-a-Pet.com, North America's largest Web-based pet-

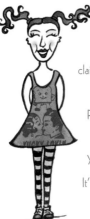

adoption service. Ms. Luwis lives and works in a historic neighborhood in northern Virginia that seems to have more dogs and cats than people. She and her boyfriend, musician Bryan Aspey, proudly support the effort, claiming one lovely rescue dog from Mexico and Bryan's beloved cat, Dorian.

Please consider adopting a pet from a shelter or rescue group. Millions of dogs and cats are euthanized every year because they do not find homes. You can search for the perfect pet at www.1-800-Save-A-Pet.com. It's FREE! It's easy! And it will help save a life! Thank you!

We'd love to hear your thoughts . . .
the good, the bad, and the not so pretty!
Email: yoga@rescuegirl.com
Web: www.rescuegirl.com
Snail mail: Box 4575, Falls Church, VA 22044